10/96

The Asthma Sourcebook

The Asthma Sourcebook

Everything You Need to Know

by Francis V. Adams, M.D.

Lowell House
Los Angeles

Contemporary Books
Chicago

Library of Congress Cataloging-in-Publication Data

Adams, Francis V.
    The asthma sourcebook : everything you need to know / by Francis V. Adams.
        p.   cm.
    Includes bibliographical references and index.
    ISBN 1-56565-329-7
    1. Asthma—Popular works.   I. Title.
RC591.A325 1995
616.2'38—dc20   95-4742
                                                                CIP

Requests for such permissions should be addressed to:
Lowell House
2029 Century Park East, Suite 3290
Los Angeles, CA 90067

Lowell House books can be purchased at special discounts when ordered in bulk for premiums and special sales. Contact Department VH at the address above.

Publisher: Jack Artenstein
General Manager, Lowell House Adult: Bud Sperry
Text Design: Susan H. Hartman

Manufactured in the United States of America
10 9 8 7 6 5 4 3 2 1

This book is dedicated to my wife, Laurie,
whose love and support are constant.

Contents

CHAPTER 4
The Asthma
Medications

CHAPTER 7
Asthma and
Pregnancy

**CHAPTER 11
Asthma and
Special
Considerations**

Figures and Tables

Until I feared I would lose it, I never loved to read. One does not love breathing.

Harper Lee
To Kill A Mockingbird

Introduction

ASTHMA is a common disease that affects nearly 5 percent of the population in the United States, perhaps as many as 13 million Americans. Since asthma is often a mild illness, these numbers probably underestimate the true number of cases. In 1990, the cost of illness related to asthma was estimated at $6.2 billion. Each year, about one million new cases are diagnosed, and this number continues to rise. Between 1982 and 1992, the asthma rate increased by 42 percent, an increase attributed partly to air pollution since the majority of asthmatics live in areas where pollution levels are high. Indoor pollution may also be a factor because windowless offices and airtight homes reduce air circulation, thus exposing asthmatics to higher levels of irritating substances.

Along with the rise in case numbers the number of deaths related to asthma has also gone up despite more and better drugs available to treat asthma. The cause of these increasing fatalities is still being debated, but several factors have already been implicated. One of the most disturbing theories suggests that overuse of a potent group of asthma drugs (the beta agonists) may be a factor in these deaths. However, many investigators feel that overuse of beta-agonists simply identifies the most severely afflicted asthmatics who are more likely to die anyway. Physicians on both sides of this debate would agree that overusing these drugs is clearly detrimental, but further research is needed to settle this crucial question.

In the last five years significant advances have improved medical science's understanding of asthma. Even the definition of asthma has changed during this period: Asthma has been re-classified as an inflammatory process. Besides greater understanding of the disease, physicians are now armed with a number of new medications they hope will improve treatment and management of asthma. An entirely new class of medication, a "mediator antagonist," will soon be available to patients in the United States.

This book aims to educate asthmatics in order to improve their quality of life. Knowledge is essential to the beneficial management of asthma. A patient must first accept the presence of the disease then take an active role in its treatment. Too often patient denial of their illness leads to more frequent and more severe asthmatic attacks. Asthma symptoms may be monitored at home, which encourages patients to participate in their own treatment. A well-informed patient is likelier to seek medical advice before an attack becomes severe. Improved communication between patients and physicians usually leads to formation of a "partnership" that helps both achieve better asthma treatment.

This book may also be helpful for friends and families of asthma patients. If others gain greater knowledge of the disease, they may be encouraged to provide vital support and better understanding.

Fatal asthma continues to occur when patients are either mistakenly diagnosed, diagnosed too late, or do not seek medical attention. These deaths are always tragic since treatment can be effective if given early and correctly. I hope this book will allow some patients to recognize they may have asthma and direct them to an appropriate care-giver. Those who have been diagnosed may learn how to better assess the degree of severity of their illness and to plan how they will respond to an attack. In this way a greater number of asthmatic attacks may be recognized and treated before they become severe or prove fatal.

All patients should seek information from their physicians. This book is meant to be used as a supplement that hopefully will add useful information. All patients should know their disease and should ask questions to increase their understanding. Appendix A contains additional suggestions for obtaining more information. In my experience some of the most useful information comes from patient-initiated discussion.

Much of the information in this book comes from listening to patients with asthma. I have also been privileged to study with a number of chest specialists who taught and encouraged me to pursue my practice of chest medicine. As a teenager I followed my father, Dr. Vincent J. Adams, on housecalls and hospital rounds and saw firsthand what being a physician meant. When I was 16 my father taught me to do pulmonary function tests as well as the basics of their interpretation which I continue to use in my own practice. At a young age I learned from him that you had to know and treat patients as individuals, not just as diseases.

When I was a medical student at Cornell Drs. James Smith and Elliot Hochstein encouraged my interest in chest disease. At Georgetown University Hospital Dr. Sol Katz embodied what a diagnostician of chest diseases should be. Finally, on the Bellevue Chest Service three of the "giants" of chest medicine, Drs. John McClement, H. William Harris and Lynn Christianson completed my formal chest education. The knowledge I gained from these gifted physicians and from nearly twenty years of "hands on" experience treating chest diseases provided the foundation for this book.

My opinions and recommendations represent my own approach to the treatment of bronchial asthma and should be so regarded. Controversies and differences of opinion permeate every aspect of medicine and asthma is no exception.

I am indebted to many for their assistance in preparing this text but can only mention a few. The medical illustrations were done by Laurel H. Adams. The photographs for Figures 5, 6, 9, 15, 16, and 17 were done by Linda Covello. Mary Kane provided many helpful suggestions as well as research and background material. Bud Sperry of Lowell House brought this project to my attention and enlisted my participation. I am grateful for that opportunity and hope this book will prove useful.

CHAPTER 1

What Is Asthma?

TO understand asthma you must first consider the normal structure of the lung. We will define asthma and discuss its causes as well as describe how a physician begins to make a diagnosis.

The Normal Lung

The Bronchial Tubes

In a normal lung, two systems coexist to permit its function of enriching the blood with oxygen and excreting carbon dioxide. Oxygen is the fuel for metabolism while carbon dioxide represents the waste product.

The first system is a series of hollow connecting airways that form the bronchial tubes. Imagine that this system resembles a large branching tree with the trunk being the windpipe (trachea) that begins below the voice box (larynx). Figure 1 shows the windpipe branching into two major bronchial divisions. Branching of this bronchial "tree" occurs frequently to the smallest imaginable airway, a bronchiole. The inner lining of the bronchial tubes is a delicate membrane called the bronchial mucosa. Although normally pale and innocent in appearance this membrane is capable of becoming inflamed and swollen in an asthmatic attack. Mucus glands within the layers of the bronchial lining can produce large quantities of extremely thick secretion when stimulated by infection or asthma triggers. In the wall of the bronchial tubes is a smooth muscle layer capable of contracting, producing narrowing or bronchoconstriction, and relaxing, producing widening or bronchodilatation.

The Alveoli

The second system within the lung consists of millions of tiny air sacs or alveoli. Think of these sacs surrounding the small bronchial tubes like grapes surrounding a stem. In Figure 2 a bronchiole is surrounded by alveoli. Each of the smallest bronchioles allows air to enter and leave multiple alveoli. Within these small air sacs the vital gas exchange takes place. Within the wall of these sacs blood courses within small vessels called capillaries. This blood has been returned from all parts of the body where it has been used for metabolism. As it enters the capillaries it is low in oxygen and high in carbon dioxide. The extremely thin walls of these blood vessels allow the exchange of oxygen and carbon dioxide. The blood leaves the alveoli oxygen rich with lower carbon dioxide levels.

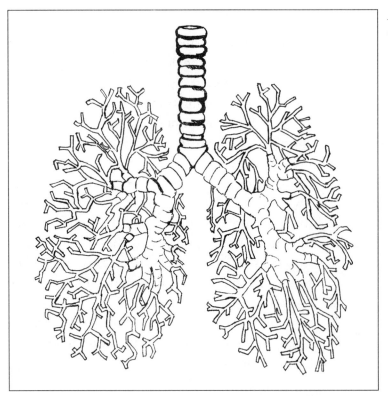

Figure 1.
The Normal Lung

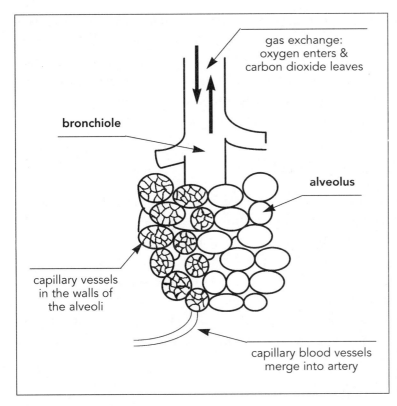

gas exchange:
oxygen enters &
carbon dioxide leaves

bronchiole

alveolus

capillary vessels
in the walls of
the alveoli

capillary blood vessels
merge into artery

Figure 2.
Bronchiole
and Alveoli

The Nervous System and the Lung

Besides reviewing the normal structure of the lung, it is important to understand the role of the nervous system and how it relates to bronchial asthma. The nervous system is generally divided into the central structures of the brain and spinal cord and peripheral nerve structures distributed throughout the body.

The Autonomic Nervous System

One major subdivision of the nervous system is called the autonomic nervous system, which is responsible for the unconscious control of major body functions and is divided into a parasympathetic and a sympathetic branch. These systems extend throughout the body but are extremely important in lung function. Just think of these two systems as balancing each other. For example, stimulating the parasympathetic system causes the bronchial tubes to constrict while stimulating the sympathetic nervous system produces the opposite reaction (dilatation). In a normal lung a balance of these two systems maintains open airways. In an asthmatic lung, an imbalance occurs favoring the parasympathetic system that produces narrowing or constriction of the air tubes.

Adrenergic Versus Cholinergic Effects

The effects produced through the nerve pathways are mediated by chemicals called neurotransmitters. These chemicals act at nerve endings or receptor sites throughout the body. In the parasympathetic nervous system the neurotransmitter is a chemical substance known as acetylcholine. Agents or medications that mimic the effects of this substance are called cholinergic agents. In the sympathetic nervous system the neurotransmitter is a substance known as epinephrine or adrenaline. Agents or medications that mimic the effects of adrenaline are called adrenergic agents.

Receptors: Alpha and Beta

It is important to familiarize yourself with the different types of receptors that exist in the nerve endings. These receptors are divided into alphas and betas based on how they respond to medication. In general, alpha receptors excite and beta receptors usually inhibit or relax. Alpha receptors seem to be less important in regulating bronchial tubes than beta receptors. Beta receptors are classified as B_1, found in the heart muscle, and B_2, found in the bronchial tubes and other parts of the body. The effect of asthma medications on these receptors is discussed in chapter 4.

Definition of Asthma

That asthma has been defined in so many ways reflects the complexity of this illness. Several features of asthma are covered by the currently accepted definition.

Airway Obstruction: Reversible

First, the airways of the lung or bronchial tubes are narrowed. This is called "airway obstruction" since air can no longer flow smoothly through this elaborate system of branching tubes. Since these tubes can dilate or open in asthma this obstruction is called reversible, an important aspect of the definition since it may distinguish asthma from other bronchial illnesses with fixed or irreversible obstruction like bronchitis and emphysema.

This narrowing within the bronchial tubes has occurred due to a tightening or constriction of the muscle that exists in the bronchial wall. This reaction may be thought of as a muscle "spasm" that results in narrowing of the bronchial tubes, similar to any muscle cramp.

It is these narrowed or "obstructed" airways that produce one of the common features of asthma, the wheeze. As air is exhaled through these tubes, its movement is turbulent and produces this sound.

Inflammation

The second element included in defining asthma is the presence of inflammation, the red, swollen appearance of the inside of the bronchial tubes. This characteristic of asthma has received a great deal of attention recently and has become the focus of much of asthma therapy. The inflammation is present in the lining (the mucosa) of the bronchial tubes, which can be examined by inserting into them a lighted scope called a bronchoscope. With this instrument a physician can also obtain samples of the bronchial lining and its secretions. Under a microscope these samples may show large numbers of cells that carry substances called mediators capable of causing inflammation. Using these techniques, the asthma mediators released by inflammatory cells when an attack occurs can be measured and identified.

Hyperirritability

The third defining feature is increased responsiveness or hyperirritability of the bronchial tubes and their tendency to "over react" and narrow. The term "twitchy" has also been used in this regard. This irritability is often demonstrated by the sudden, severe attacks patients can experience when exposed to substances such as pollen, animal dander, dust, and fumes. This hyperreactivity forms the basis for bronchial provocation or challenge testing that is used by physicians to diagnose asthma in patients whose illnesses do not fit easily into the other definitions.

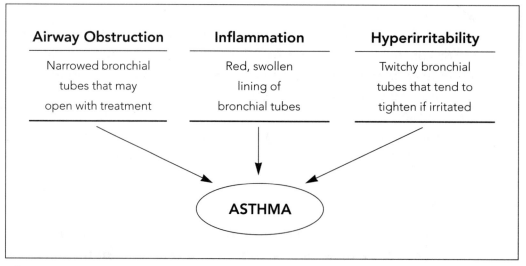

Figure 3.
Definition of Asthma

What Causes Asthma?

Although asthma may be defined by the factors noted above, its cause remains uncertain. At this time it appears several factors are involved.

Heredity

Heredity certainly plays a major role: asthma and allergy often occur in families. Geneticists have located a gene on chromosome 11 that is strongly associated with allergy and speculate that several other genes may also be involved. One study suggests that a variant gene may direct the immune system to "overreact" to allergic stimuli by allowing a protein known as Immunoglobulin E (IgE) to "lock on" to the surface of allergy cells called mast cells. When IgE reacts with allergy substances known as allergens, the mast cell disintegrates, releasing irritating chemicals that cause inflammation. These chemicals are the asthma mediators. Further research will undoubtedly produce a more detailed explanation for the genetic basis of asthma.

The Immune System

The immune system also plays a major role in the development of asthma. The immune system has two basic branches: cellular and humoral. Cellular immunity involves white blood cells called lymphocytes that can be provoked or "sensitized." An example of this would be the body's rejection process against a transplanted organ. Humoral immunity involves production of substances called antibodies that circulate in the blood. An example would be how the body reacts to a vaccination by producing antibodies. An antigen (may be called an allergen) is a substance capable of provoking the immune response.

Lymphocytes, Mast Cells, and Eosinophils

In asthma, the immune system is provoked in two ways. First, the cellular elements are mobilized and activated. Microscopic studies of the lining of the bronchial tubes in asthma have revealed increased numbers of lymphocytes. These cells produce substances that result in an increase in the number of mast cells that are known to store and release many irritating chemicals involved in production of the asthmatic reaction. These chemical substances or mediators of asthma produce inflammation. Another active cell that is "recruited" by lymphocytes found in the inflamed bronchial lining is the eosinophil. Large numbers of these cells may also be found in the blood of allergic and asthmatic individuals.

Immunoglobulin E

The second major immune response in asthma is the production of antibodies known as immunoglobulins, which is stimulated by substances released by the activated lymphocytes. One type, Immunoglobulin E or

IgE, may be produced by inhaling a specific foreign substance such as rag-weed. When the IgE attaches to the surface of the mast cell, a process is initiated that leads to release of the "asthma chemicals" and an ensuing asthmatic reaction.

Allergy

Allergy is the leading cause of asthma. In many patients allergens, activated lymphocytes, mast cells, eosinophils, and IgE all play major roles in the immune response that produces the asthmatic reaction. However, asthma may also occur without allergy. In non-allergic patients doctors believe the immune response may be triggered by infection.

Viruses

Viral infections in susceptible individuals have been thought to be potent triggers for the development of asthma. Animal research has shown that viruses are capable of altering the nervous impulses that stimulate the bronchial tubes. The altered nerve impulses may then produce constriction in the bronchial tubes. Susceptible patients with viral bronchial infections may become "sensitized" and display all the features noted in the definition of asthma.

The Environment

Environmental irritants, such as cigarette smoke, pollutants (ozone, particulates), dust, and chemicals and proteins found in the home and the workplace are also considered capable of provoking the asthmatic response. These irritants may account for large numbers of asthmatic attacks each year and may also, in part, explain an increase in the number of asthma cases.

The Nervous System

Another possible cause of asthma is a dysfunction of nerve receptors or endings in the muscle surrounding the bronchial tubes that produces con-

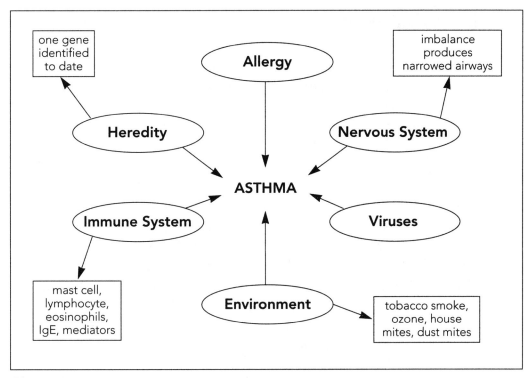

Figure 4.
Causes of Asthma

striction of the air passage. Research has shown that an imbalance may exist in the nervous system that supplies the bronchial tubes of asthmatic individuals. This inborn error may shift the balance of forces toward those nerve signals that promote narrowing of the bronchial passages.

The Future

At this time the specific causes of asthma and the signals that are involved in starting the chain reaction that produces the disease are unknown. In the last five years promising research has shown that asthma is an inflammatory disease with features similar to other illnesses such as arthritis. This breakthrough is likely to lead to a further understanding of the causes of asthma and will likely form the basis for greater advances in treatment.

Extrinsic Versus Intrinsic Asthma

Asthma is often divided into either an allergic or "extrinsic" type that commonly has its onset in childhood, and an adult-onset or "intrinsic" type. Although there is considerable overlap between these groups it is helpful to classify patients according to several features that distinguish them.

Extrinsic Asthma

Extrinsic patients are younger and have attacks clearly triggered by exposure to allergens like pollens, dust, animal dander, foods, and molds. These patients often have strong family histories of relatives with allergies or asthma. Allergy treatment known as desensitization has often been helpful in these patients. For many years it has been thought that the majority of these patients "outgrew" their asthma by age thirty but recent evidence suggests that 75 percent remain asthmatic for life. These patients may have long symptom-free periods.

Intrinsic Asthma

Intrinsic group patients often develop asthma as adults, and at any age. Often the trigger for these attacks is infection with involvement of the lower respiratory tract as in bronchitis or pneumonia. Some of the most severe infections of this type are viral but may also be bacterial. Patients in the intrinsic group usually do not have histories of allergies and produce negative allergy tests. Once the diagnosis is evident further attacks are often triggered by less severe infections. There are fewer symptom-free periods in this group and these patients usually require medication for life.

Should this Classification Be Used?

Many practitioners no longer use this older classification of the types of bronchial asthma. When discussing the future outlook of the disease as well as treatment options, I find it helpful to use these two general classes of asthma to provide simple guidelines that can be followed. In the younger, highly allergic or extrinsic asthmatic, for example, emphasis on avoidance of allergens will be extremely important. Less time would be spent discussing this topic for patients with intrinsic asthma.

How Is the Diagnosis of Asthma Made?

The Medical History

All diagnosis begins with a thorough medical history. The physician looks for the age at onset of symptoms and associated allergies. Evidence of airway obstruction may be suggested by a report of wheezing and shortness of breath. Coughing may be a prominent symptom and the physician will inquire as to the character of phlegm produced. The physician will also ask about the presence of nasal symptoms or sinus pain or infection as well as the presence of allergic skin problems such as rash (eczema) or hives (urticaria). A diminished sense of smell or taste may suggest the presence of nasal polyps. Common questions include: "What seems to trigger your attack?" "What are your attacks like?" Asthma often worsens at night and the patient may be asked "Do you ever awaken with an attack?" The timing of attacks other than at night is also important. A relationship between asthma and hormonal influences should be explored. Many women note increased asthmatic symptoms before their period as well as changes during pregnancy. The physician will ask about the effect of exercise on the patient's symptoms since asthma may occasionally occur only with exercise. Emotional factors will also be investigated as potential triggers. "Are you under more stress?" A thorough family history will also be obtained since the presence of asthma or allergy in closely related family members will support the diagnosis. The physician will also ask about occupation and possible exposures to irritating chemicals, dust, or fumes. To help establish the hyperresponsiveness evident in asthma the physician will ask how the patient reacts to changes in temperature, humidity, air pollution, or the presence of cigarette smoke, fumes or odors. Reaction to foods containing sulfites as well as to drugs (especially aspirin and penicillin) are also important historical factors.

Looking for Asthma Triggers

When obtaining the initial history the physician must be like a detective, especially in examining sources of irritation that may have precipitated or irritated an underlying asthmatic condition. Both the home and workplace must be reviewed in that context. Many patients are aware of the "sick building syndrome" in which asthma may be produced by a particular contaminant and thus are able to give important information. The type of heating and cooling system in place should be known. Although the patient may be a nonsmoker sources of secondhand smoke should be investigated. "Have you recently moved or renovated?" "Do you have pets?" "How often do you clean your humidifier?" If attacks occur frequently at night the bedroom should be singled out for review. "Do you have a mattress cover?" "What type of floor covering do you have?"

It is not unusual for a patient to supply information that may identify a specific source of irritation and asthma attacks. A 34-year-old man was referred to me for asthma that was extremely difficult to control. He had had many severe attacks and was receiving several asthma medications. Corticosteroids had been prescribed several times and he had noted side effects of weight gain and stomach upset. The patient noted that he was often well during the day but worsened at night, especially after returning to his apartment. The patient often worked in his bedroom where he spent a great deal of time when he was home. He was often awakened during the night by wheezing and shortness of breath and noted that he was "worse in the morning." Asthma attacks often occurred whenever he attempted to clean his apartment. I suspected he was allergic to dust mites and that was confirmed by allergy testing. The patient acquired a mattress cover and began following several recommendations mentioned in chapter 6. He returned for a visit after six weeks and noted he was now sleeping through the night and awakening without wheezing. His medications were sharply reduced and he has not required further corticosteroids. I often remind him that the credit for his improvement belongs to his mattress cover.

Participating in Your Care

Patients can be extremely helpful by detailing that type of specific information for the physician. Write down the important facts in your history that you want to present to your physician. If this narrative is lengthy, send the material ahead of you with other medical records so your physician can review it in detail before your visit. You can be an active participant in your care. Start at the initial interview with your physician. The more detailed information you can supply, particularly in the areas noted above, the more accurate the diagnosis will be. It is also helpful to describe to your physician how your symptoms have affected your life at home and at work. It is extremely helpful for your physician to know what kind of support you as a patient can rely on as well as whether there are any adverse influences in your life, either environmental or emotional. Reviewing this material is time-consuming and addressing the relief of asthma may take precedent, so tell your physician you want to discuss certain topics at another time. Use a portion of each office visit to discuss a specific topic.

Too often patients are treated only when severe asthmatic symptoms emerge, often requiring emergency room care. While this is essential and often lifesaving the "quick fix" of ER treatment is not designed for the careful historical review needed to make the correct diagnosis of asthma.

The Physical Examination

The next step in diagnosis of asthma is the physical examination, where your physician seeks to correlate the historical information you have provided. For example, the skin and nasal passages are examined for allergic manifestations such as eczema and rhinitis. In the nose, the finding of nasal polyps identifies the patient as someone who may have severe asthma or allergy.

Examination of the chest is extremely important. The physician will note the quality of the breath sounds as air is inhaled and exhaled. When there is airway obstruction the flow of air through the bronchial tubes is turbulent and often creates wheezing, which is more commonly noted upon exhaling. In addition, the narrowed passages prolong the time it takes for air to be exhaled and the physician will note a prolonged expiratory phase. Although the patient's breathing may be quiet at rest, when asked to take a deep breath and exhale, wheezing and cough may then occur. This maneuver enables a physician to discover an airway obstruction.

Asthma Without Wheezing ('Cough Asthma')

In the last several years it has become clear that a group of patients with all the characteristics of asthma (airway obstruction, inflammation and hyperresponsiveness) may never manifest wheezing. In these patients a persistent cough is the main symptom. Although the physical exam may be unremarkable these patients often have typical histories of cough attacks at night or triggered by exposure to allergens. Laboratory evaluation will often demonstrate all the features of asthma. This syndrome is often identified as the "asthma equivalent syndrome" or "cough asthma." In the past too much weight has been put on the presence of wheezing in the diagnosis of asthma.

Wheezing Without Asthma

Just as the absence of wheezing has often led to patients being misdiagnosed as nonasthmatic, the presence of wheezing also may lead to the erroneous diagnosis of asthma. It has been said that "all that wheezes is not asthma" since many illnesses may produce turbulent airflow through the airways. Too often patients are "diagnosed" simply on this one physical finding.

Wheezing may occur in a variety of illnesses, such as when lesions produce a fixed blockage or obstruction in an air passage. In a child or an adult this may be as simple as a foreign body that has been aspirated. In these cases wheezing may be localized to one area or one lung, which should alert the physician to such a possibility. The history of onset may have been sudden, following a "choking spell." In an adult with a history of smoking a lung tumor that may be benign or malignant may also produce wheezing by growing within the bronchial tube and blocking the airflow. In these and similar cases, chest x-rays and diagnostic techniques like bronchoscopy often produce the correct diagnosis.

Emphysema and Chronic Bronchitis

Many respiratory illnesses are characterized by wheezing and may be mistaken for asthma. Emphysema is a disease in which the elasticity of the lung is reduced often resulting in closure of the airways. The term "floppy airways" is often used in this disease to describe how easily the bronchial tubes may close and produce wheezing. Chronic bronchitis is a disease in which there is chronic cough and mucus production. Wheezing is often produced by the clogged and inflamed airways of these patients.

Cystic Fibrosis and Bronchiectasis

Patients with cystic fibrosis, a genetic deficiency disease occurring in children and young adults, often have wheezing due to the clogging of their bronchial tubes by an abnormally viscous mucus. A similar mechanism explains the wheezing found in patients with bronchiectasis, an illness in which infections have permanently damaged the bronchial tubes leading to plugging and inflammation.

Heart Failure ('Cardiac Asthma')

In patients with heart failure fluid may collect in the lungs around or within the bronchial tubes. These patients often complain of wheezing, especially at night, mimicking the asthma patient. Due to these similar features this has been called "cardiac asthma" although it is a heart syndrome that often resolves with mobilization of the lung fluid by specific medication. The diagnosis is often made by additional physical findings of heart disease as well as by the chest x-ray and other tests of heart function.

Laryngeal Asthma

A rare but increasingly reported illness that produces wheezing and may be misdiagnosed as asthma is vocal cord dysfunction syndrome. This syndrome is also known as "laryngeal asthma" since in this illness wheezing is produced at the voice box by an abnormal closure of the vocal cords when the patient breathes in (inspiration). Normally, the vocal cords separate on inspiration allowing more air to flow into the lungs. In these patients the sounds of turbulent flow are transmitted over the lung fields mimicking the wheezing of asthma. The cause of this disorder is unknown. It is thought to be involuntary and often responds to voice therapy. The diagnosis may only be made by direct visualization of the vocal cords by the physician. This is increasingly done with a fiberoptic scope. Pulmonary function testing (see chapter 2) may also suggest this diagnosis.

The Next Step

Up to this point the physician has used his interview techniques to obtain an accurate history and his physical diagnostic skills to form a working diagnosis of bronchial asthma. In order to confirm that impression, laboratory testing and especially pulmonary function testing will be required. These techniques will be discussed in chapter 2.

CHAPTER 2

Laboratory Evaluation of Asthma

FOLLOWING the careful review of the patient's history and physical examination the physician will proceed to several commonly used laboratory tests to complete the diagnostic evaluation. There is no universal "checklist" of tests for every patient since there is great variation in each case. Physicians may also have differences in their laboratory evaluations.

Blood Tests

In the laboratory evaluation of asthma it would be common to evaluate the patient's blood count looking for "allergy cells" called eosinophils. The physician may also obtain a level of IgE, the immunoglobulin in the blood that is often elevated in allergic patients.

X-Rays

A chest x-ray is often necessary to exclude many of the entities discussed above that can mimic asthma. It does not serve to confirm the diagnosis since the features of asthma occurring within the bronchial tubes cannot be seen on a chest x-ray.

Occasionally, the chest x-ray may show that the lungs are greatly expanded and appear larger than normal or hyperinflated. This occurs in asthma because air may enter the bronchial tubes but have difficulty being exhaled, also known as "air-trapping." This x-ray finding cannot be used as a diagnostic tool for asthma since the same finding may occur in emphysema and in some cases of bronchitis.

Often the physician will order sinus x-rays as part of the laboratory evaluation. Evidence of sinusitis or nasal polyps would identify patients as high-risk candidates for asthma. In addition, the sinusitis may be viewed as a potential aggravating factor in asthmatic attacks and thus become a focus of treatment of individual patients. There is a recent trend toward using the more detailed CAT scan for this exam because of the increased information it provides.

Sputum Exam

Examination of swabs of nasal mucus or chest phlegm (sputum) may be helpful in diagnosing asthma. Microscopic examination may identify abundant eosinophils that would be characteristic of allergy and asthma. The presence of pus cells called neutrophils would suggest an infectious process, i.e. bronchitis or sinusitis. The physician may request a culture of the coughed sputum if pus cells are seen under the microscope.

Pulmonary Function Testing

Forced Expiratory Maneuver

The most important laboratory test the physician performs in the diagnosis of asthma is pulmonary function testing. Before the testing begins the patient's age, race, sex, height, and weight are recorded. From these statistics the expected normal values are determined. These are called the predicted normals and they are determined from statistical analysis of large groups of normal subjects.

The most common test involves a device known as a spirometer, which measures the amount of air (volume) expelled by the patient as well as its speed as the air is exhaled forcefully. In this simple but extremely important maneuver the patient is asked to take a full deep breath in then exhale fully and forcefully—*this is called a maximum forced expiratory maneuver*. In tracing this maneuver the physician determines the maximum amount of air the patient can expel after the deepest inhalation. This amount is called the vital capacity. Figure 5 shows a patient performing pulmonary function testing.

As air is expelled the airflow is measured throughout the maneuver until the patient is unable to exhale further. One extremely useful measurement is of the greatest flow that can be obtained after the patient has inhaled fully and forcefully exhaled. This is termed peak expiratory flow rate or "peak flow." This important and easily performed measurement will be discussed in chapter 3. Flow rates are recorded at the beginning, middle and end of the forced exhalation maneuver and so is the amount of air expelled each second. As air is exhaled by the lungs it is the large bronchial tubes (large airways) that empty first with the smaller passages (small airways) contributing a greater share as exhalation continues and ends. In one second a certain amount of air should normally be exhaled with an expected increase as time increases. The one second measurement is often a good reflector of the large airways and measurements toward the middle and end of the breath usually determine the condition of smaller air passages.

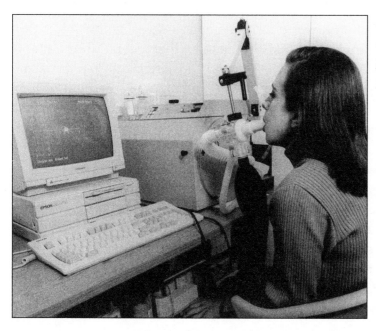

Figure 5. Performing pulmonary function tests

Evaluating the Effect of Asthma Medication

Since asthma has been defined as an illness characterized in part by airway obstruction it is essential for diagnosis to demonstrate this by using spirometry. The definition also includes the feature of reversibility, that is, that airflow can improve significantly. To demonstrate this feature spirometry is performed before and after inhaling bronchodilator medication. To be significant, the physician looks for at least a 15 percent improvement in the spirometry parameters after the patient inhales bronchodilator medication.

Diseases such as emphysema, chronic bronchitis, cystic fibrosis, or bronchiectasis may demonstrate severe degrees of airflow obstruction without any improvement after bronchodilator use. However, it may be difficult to demonstrate reversibility in all asthmatics during a single laboratory session, possibly owing to severe degrees of bronchial narrowing or to inadequate inhalation of medication by the patient. Therefore, the absence of reversibility should never be taken as absolute proof that asthma is not present.

Further Testing

Besides simple spirometry, the physician may perform other pulmonary function tests to better assess and define a patient's condition. Patients with a variety of illnesses may have reduced capacities and flow rates and further testing may be needed. These tests include measurement of lung volume in which the different divisions or "compartments" of the lungs are measured. These divisions represent quantities of air that are distributed throughout the lung. One example would be the quantity of air that remains in the lung at all times to keep it expanded.

Measuring of lung volumes may be performed by two methods. A common technique requires inhaling a special gas mixture containing helium that the patient breathes for several minutes. Analyzing the amount of helium exhaled allows the physician to calculate how the air was distributed in the different air divisions of the lung. Another technique for measuring lung volumes requires an airtight box called a body plethysmograph. In this technique the patient sits in a clear box that resembles a phone booth and breathes against a mouthpiece. By analyzing pressure changes in the box as the patient breathes it is possible to determine the volume of gas in the lungs.

Another important pulmonary function test is known as a diffusion capacity. This is a sensitive test for the loss of gas exchanging units of the lung as in emphysema. These units are the air sacs or alveoli described in chapter 1. In this test the patient again breathes a special gas mixture and an amount of exhaled gas is collected. By determining how fast the inhaled gas has disappeared, it is possible to determine whether the air sacs are exchanging gases normally.

Exercise Testing

The above tests are performed with the patient at rest. Since exercise may create narrowing of the airways an exercise test may be extremely helpful in demonstrating that a patient develops asthma with exercise or that a patient with mild disease has worse airflow parameters after exercise. Such a test may be performed with a treadmill or a stationary bicycle. The patient is asked to slowly increase the level of exercise until either a certain heart rate is achieved or shortness of breath develops. At this point the patient is asked to perform spirometry and the airflows are compared to those obtained prior to exercise. If the exercise produces significant narrowing of the air tubes, the flow rates will be lower, confirming an asthmatic response. This procedure usually requires less than 10 minutes of exercise and is performed under close observation.

Bronchial Challenge Testing

A challenge test may be used by the physician to demonstrate that a patient with a normal result on pulmonary function testing may indeed have asthma. This bronchial challenge or provocation testing would only be performed if the patient's history and physical findings suggested that the patient is asthmatic but spirometry was normal. It is not a routine part of pulmonary function testing. The substances or agents commonly used for challenge testing include histamine, methacholine, and cold air.

Histamine is stored in allergy cells such as mast cells and is released during allergic or asthmatic attacks. It is thought to be one of the media-tors of asthma. For this reason it is very suitable for provoking asthma in challenge testing. Methacholine is a chemical that stimulates one part of the nervous system called the parasympathetic nervous system to fire. If inhaled into the bronchial tubes in an asthmatic subject, methacholine will trigger impulses that produce airway constriction. Cold air irritates the bronchial tubes and may also be used for challenge testing. In an asth-matic subject with hyperreactive airways, inhaling cold air will produce significant tightening of the bronchial tubes.

In the patient thought to have occupational asthma the specific offend-ing substance may be used to confirm the direct link between the sub-stance and the patient's asthmatic reaction. A similar challenge test has been used in patients to confirm allergy to sulfites and aspirin. With any challenge test there is a risk of a severe asthmatic reaction and for this reason these tests are reserved for difficult diagnostic situations and are only performed under careful observation and control.

Guidelines have been developed for performing and interpreting bronchial challenge testing. It is vital to standardize this type of testing to avoid "false positive" or "false negative" results. Generally, for a provoca-tion test to be positive, there must be at least a 15 percent fall in airflow after inhaling the challenge material.

Testing Oxygen Levels

Assessing enrichment of the blood with oxygen by the lung can be made by a non-invasive technique called oximetry, in which a sensor placed on the fingertip or earlobe can accurately measure oxygen saturation. Such a sensor is often immediately placed on an asthmatic patient who has been admitted to an emergency room. Oxygen saturation testing measures how much oxygen the blood has acquired in the air sacs of the lungs.

The oximeter transmits different wavelengths of light through small blood vessels called capillaries. The fingernail and earlobe are used since these small vessels are close to the surface of the skin. In these small blood vessels oxygen is carried by a protein called hemoglobin. As oxygen is used by the body, the hemoglobin undergoes a change that can be detected by a different absorption of light from the oximeter. This determination is made during each pulse beat and from the relative amounts of hemoglobin with and without oxygen, the saturation is determined. The patient's pulse is also recorded. Figure 6 shows the pulse oximeter in use.

This technique can be extremely helpful in evaluating bronchial asthma since oxygen levels will typically fall with significant degrees of airway obstruction. An asthma attack that reduces oxygen levels signifies a more severe episode and calls for aggressive medical treatment. Oximetry is painless and does not require blood sampling.

Arterial Blood Gases

A more accurate and revealing although more invasive test of gas exchange by the lung is called an arterial blood gas. In this test, blood is obtained from an artery (commonly the radial artery at the wrist) allowing a more accurate test of not only the oxygen level but carbon dioxide. Carbon dioxide (CO_2) is the waste product of the body excreted by the lungs. Severe degrees of lung disease, including asthma, can impair gas exchange mechanisms to the point that levels of CO_2 will rise. In bronchial asthma this finding identifies an extremely severe and serious attack that requires hospitalization. These patients will also have lowered oxygen levels and may require mechanical respiratory assistance.

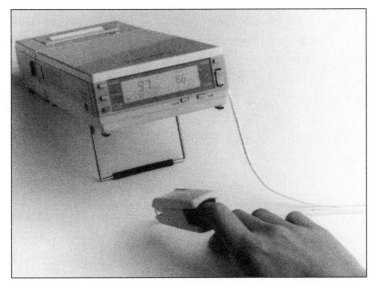

Figure 6.
Pulse oximeter

Allergy Evaluation: Is It Necessary?

As a rule, all patients with bronchial asthma should have an allergy evaluation. In children, allergy clearly plays a significant role in the severity of the disease and the frequency of attacks. In adults, the role of allergy is less important although most patients, when tested, are found to be allergic.

Allergy Skin Tests

Although useful as a screening test the IgE level by itself is not sufficient to determine the presence of allergy (also called atopy). Additional evaluation may include allergy skin testing for specific substances known as allergens that may trigger asthma attacks. This method has been used for more than 100 years and represents an extremely reliable way of determining the presence of allergy to a specific substance. Skin testing is performed by pricking, scratching, or injecting the skin with a small amount of allergen. Positive reactions, which resemble hives, are noted in 20–30 minutes. But skin testing is time consuming and may cause total body reactions in highly sensitive individuals.

Allergy Blood Tests

Evidence for allergy may also be obtained through blood testing that detects the presence of specific antibodies to various allergens. One technique is known as RAST (Radioallergosorbent test). This test utilizes radioactive material and detects the presence of a specific IgE antibody that has been produced against a certain allergen. This method is thought to be less accurate than skin testing, however, although it may prove useful in selected individuals. Other drawbacks include greater cost when compared to skin testing as well as a delay of up to 3 weeks in obtaining results.

A relatively new technique known as MAST (Multiple Antigen Simultaneous Testing) has been developed for measuring allergen-specific IgE antibodies. This technique is faster and less expensive than RAST and provides accurate results when compared to RAST and skin prick tests. Results may be obtained in one week.

Allergic Reaction

A positive allergy test does not always identify a significant allergy, so the patient's history becomes an extremely important factor in correlating allergy test results with true triggers of asthma attacks.

Immediate and 'Late' Reactions

Allergy reactions are often immediate and severe as in the patient who is allergic to bee venom, but an allergic reaction may not always be immediately apparent. Recently, it has been demonstrated that a "late phase" response may occur several hours after exposure to an offending substance. In the late phase reaction, inflammation plays a significant role and it is essential that effective therapy be directed at this component as well as to bronchial obstruction. If not treated this late phase reaction may form the basis of recurrent and increasingly severe asthma attacks.

Allergy Treatment: Avoidance and Immunotherapy

Once specific allergens have been identified, the patient must attempt to avoid these substances and clear them from home and workplace as much as possible. A natural extension of the identification of allergy is the consideration of desensitization or immunotherapy by an allergy specialist. Allergy "shots" are given after sensitivity to specific allergens have been identified. These injections contain extremely small amounts of the allergen which is slowly increased in amount. These injections produce a "blocking antibody" that interrupts the allergy reaction. Studies of immunotherapy in asthmatics have shown a reduction in symptoms and inhibition of the late asthmatic response. The administration of immunotherapy is a gradual process often requiring weeks or months to achieve a response. In older subjects the response to treatment may not be as pronounced as in younger patients. Extremely sensitive patients may experience generalized allergic reactions to the administration of allergens.

Recent studies have focused on fatal reactions to allergy injections. The majority of these cases were patients with severe asthma who had histories of severe asthmatic attacks that required steroids and hospitalization. These patients also appeared to be highly sensitive individuals who may have had a previous reaction to allergen injection.

Who Should Be Treated?

In patients with mild or moderate asthma who are well controlled on medication, allergy injections or immunotherapy should not be necessary. Those patients who are unstable should be considered candidates for treatment. In those allergic patients who are more severe or require frequent or continuous administration of corticosteroids the potential benefits of immunotherapy should be weighed against the potential for severe reactions. Once a response to immunotherapy is obtained the patient may remain on maintenance therapy for several years.

After the Diagnosis Is Made

After using these laboratory methods to confirm the diagnosis of bronchial asthma, the physician will begin to work closely with the patient to prevent asthmatic attacks. In order for this "working partnership" of physician and patient to be successful, it is necessary to understand the nature of the attack. The asthmatic attack and how it may be recognized before it becomes severe will be discussed in chapter 3.

The Asthmatic Attack

The Asthmatic Attack

AN asthmatic attack is one of the most striking medical emergencies. One of my first experiences with severe asthma was in the intensive care unit of Bellevue Hospital. I had been called to consult on a 56-year-old woman who was having a severe asthmatic attack. As I entered the unit and approached the bedside, I noted several physicians already in attendance. The patient was sitting upright with labored breathing and I could hear her wheezing from several feet away. It was clear that she was not doing well despite continuous oxygen and medicated aerosol treatment. Unable to speak due to shortness of breath, her expression was one of fear and desperation. Several days later, greatly improved after vigorous treatment, I asked her to describe what she had been feeling during her attack. "It was like I was drowning."

In the asthmatic attack there is constriction or tightening of the bronchial wall muscle, secretion of mucus often with "plugging" of small air tubes as well as inflammation and swelling of the bronchial lining. The end result is blockage or obstruction of the bronchial tubes. The frequency, duration, and severity of the asthmatic attack varies markedly from patient to patient.

Symptoms and Signs of An Attack

Although there are differences from patient to patient, the asthma attack is typically characterized by shortness of breath and wheezing. Cough and

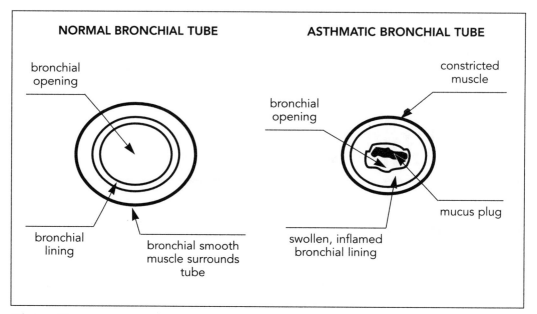

Figure 7.
Comparison of normal and asthmatic bronchial tubes

mucus production may be prominent symptoms. In some patients wheezing may not occur and a cough may be the dominant symptom. The patient demonstrates rapid rate of breathing, often with heaving of the chest and use of neck muscles to assist each breath. During an attack the patient is totally disabled. Even speech may be impossible due to severe breathlessness. The patient may be totally consumed by the effort to breathe and unable to eat or dress. The patient is often restless and unable to lie flat. Severe attacks may end in exhaustion, with ominous slowing of the respiratory rate and arrest of breathing.

Depending on the severity of the patient's disease the attack may be totally or partially reversible, allowing the patient to assume normal activities between episodes. Patients with severe asthma, however, may remain to some degree symptomatic at all times.

It should be noted that the degree of wheezing can be misleading. The severity of the asthmatic attack should never be judged on this basis alone. Some patients who are capable of moving large amounts of air may produce more turbulence and audible wheezing than others who are so severely obstructed that their breaths are shallow and incapable of producing much sound.

How to Recognize the Asthmatic Attack

Peak Flow Meter

In bronchial asthma it is extremely important to recognize the presence of an attack before it becomes severe and requires emergency measures. Each patient should have a means of assessing the degree of asthma that is present from day to day. In this manner severe episodes and often the use of oral or injectable corticosteroids necessary for such emergencies can be avoided. As an extension of this home monitoring the patient should be instructed how to respond to the presence of increased asthma. In this way a contingency plan can be in place and ready before severe attacks occur and require emergency room care. The cornerstone of this home monitoring is the peak flow meter. In essence it is an "early warning" device for individuals with asthma.

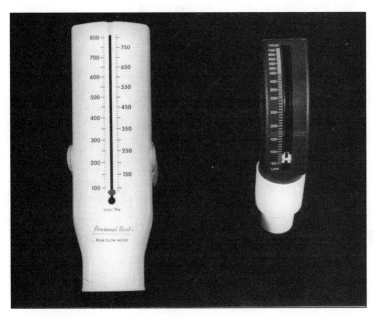

Figure 8.
Peak flow meters

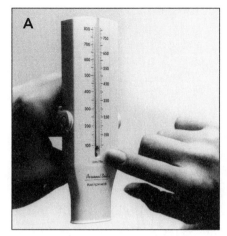

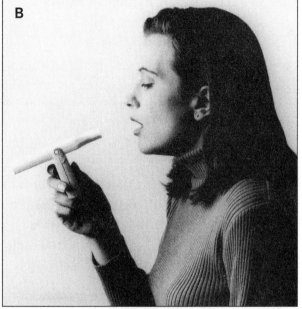

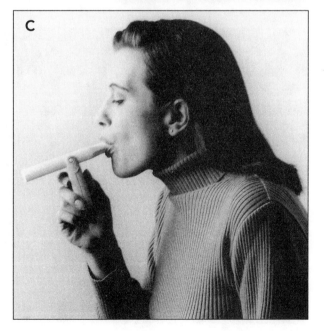

Figure 9.
Performing peak flow
measurement:
A (above)   First set meter to
            zero
B (right)   Then take a deep
            breath in . . .
C (below)   Then blow out as
            hard as you can!

What the Peak Flow Meter Measures

The peak flow meter is a simple and inexpensive device that can be used in and out of the home to monitor bronchial asthma and similar conditions. This compact device determines the maximal expiratory flow rate that the patient is capable of producing. Similar to the office spirometry the patient inhales fully and then exhales fully and forcefully into the flow meter device. A simple scale registers the peak flow. Two peak flow meters are shown in Figure 8. If done as instructed this flow rate correlates well with other measurement of airflow through the large airways of the lung. With a diary to record readings the patient can maintain an accurate assessment of the degree of asthma from day to day. This is not unlike the diabetic who records blood sugar readings. This information can be invaluable to the physician in managing patients with bronchial asthma since it gives an objective measurement to go by instead of trying to assess asthma by the degree of shortness of breath or wheezing. Communication with the physician can be much more meaningful with a record of the patient's peak flows resulting in earlier and better treatment. With earlier recognition of an attack through peak flow measurements, severe and potentially fatal asthma attacks may be avoided.

Asthma with Normal Peak Flows

Remember that peak flow measurements reflect primarily large airways and therefore do not totally assess the asthmatic condition. Normal peak flows may occur in the presence of significant small airways disease that requires continued and effective treatment. This explains why patients may continue to be symptomatic even with normal peak flow rates.

How Do I Perform a Peak Flow Measurement?

It is extremely important that peak flows be obtained in the same manner each time so that they can be compared. The meter itself should first be inspected to see that the scale indicator has been returned to zero. The patient should either sit or stand with good posture, inhale as deeply as possible (maximal inspiration) and then place the meter in the mouth with lips closed around and exhale fully and forcefully (maximal expiration). A scale records the result. I suggest performing the maneuver three times and recording the best result. Figure 9 shows a patient correctly performing the peak flow measurement. Figure 10 is an example of a peak flow diary in which readings are recorded.

Obtaining Your Personal Best Value

Once the patient has obtained and begun to use a peak flow meter it is helpful to record their "personal best effort." This result can be used as a reference value to determine if the patient's asthma is stable, improving, or deteriorating.

How Often Should I Do My Peak Flow ?

Peak flows are best if they are performed at approximately the same time each day, preferably morning and night since asthma may worsen at night. When the peak flow meter is first obtained the patient may gain information that is useful by performing flow before and after medication to determine how this influences their "personal best."

Using Peak Flows for Diagnosis

Peak flows may also have diagnostic value. Patients may be helped by determining the change in flow in different environmental settings. For example, those who often develop symptoms at work may perform flows at home and work and find that the change in environment produces decreased flows. Investigation of the offending environment may reveal the presence of allergens or pollutants that can be eliminated. Consistently lower flow in a patient's bedroom may suggest that dust mites are in great concentration. A simple remedy may be a pillow and mattress cover.

Another diagnostic test that patients may perform is determining peak flows before and after exercise. Although a formal exercise test performed in the physician's office is usually needed to diagnose exercise-induced

PEAK FLOW CHART								
	Date	Date	Date	Date	Date	Date	Date	Date
Peak Flow								
700								
600								
500								
400								
300								
200								
100								

Figure 10.
Sample of peak flow diary in which patients should record
their daily peak flow.

asthma (EIA), or to demonstrate that patients with established asthma may worsen with exercise, the patient can often gain useful information with the small, portable peak flow meter.

How Should I Interpret Changes in My Peak Flow?

The greatest value of the peak flow meter is as an "early warning" system for the patient's bronchial asthma. It is important to first establish your normal or "personal best" value. From large numbers of volunteers predicted normal values are available for reference. It should be noted that the patient's normal may not equal what is predicted and it is best to use peak flow results in reference to the patient's best result. Flow is expressed as liters per minute (l/min).

Using the Reference Value

If your best peak flow has been 300 l/min, this should be the reference value you would consider your "normal" result. This may increase with treatment and therefore the higher value will become the reference value. Peak flows vary with sex, age, and body size. Remember that peak flow will vary with effort. If a less than maximal effort is given then falsely low readings will be obtained. This is why the patient should always try to perform the peak flow measurement in the same way and why three efforts should be performed each time.

Interpreting Drops in Peak Flow

When asthmatic attacks occur peak flows drop due to constriction of the airways. For the patient with a personal best of 400 l/min, a drop of 50 percent to 200 l/min indicates a severe attack and the need for aggressive treatment. The value of the peak flow meter is also its ability to detect less severe drops in flow that allow the patient to administer treatment as outlined by the physician. Therefore a decrease of 25 percent to 300 l/min identifies a mild to moderate attack. If appropriate treatment is given at this time then a severe attack may be avoided. Treatment at this point may not include the use of corticosteroids whereas more severe attacks will commonly require steroid use.

When Your Peak Flow Is Normal

Peak flow measurements may be helpful in a positive way. Shortness of breath may occur from a variety of sources, including anxiety. Patients with severe breathlessness who obtain normal peak flows may benefit greatly from this positive reinforcement and may then focus on other possible sources of this symptom other than asthma.

Why Not Do Peak Flows?

Although a peak flow meter is extremely inexpensive and requires only a few seconds to use, peak flows are often not done. A 46-year-old woman who has frequent asthmatic attacks often calls for instructions during a severe episode. I can usually hear wheezing over the phone and recognize from her speech pattern that she is short of breath. When I ask for her record of peak flows she states that "I haven't been doing it lately but I'll try to do one now." She registers 100 l/min and is instructed to proceed to the nearest emergency room. This usually results in the use of corticosteroids which may have been avoided if the attack had been recognized earlier.

Unfortunately, this conversation is repeated several times a week with patients who have had severe asthmatic attacks. In many individuals the failure to use a peak flow meter despite severe asthma is one indicator of who may suffer a fatal attack. In my experience these patients often do not take their medications as directed. Frequently, this behavior appears to result from denial. Many patients do not accept that they have asthma and that it is a chronic disease that requires regular monitoring and medication. Only through patient education and counseling can denial be overcome.

A 60-year-old man with asthma had just finished providing me with his medical history. "I also want you to know that I have a lovely wife and grandchildren and that your job is to keep me alive so I can enjoy them! What can I do to help myself?" A long conversation followed but I can assure you that it included the use of a peak flow meter.

Home or the Emergency Room?

Having a Treatment Plan

The drop in peak flow to 50 percent of the patient's best identifies a serious attack. The patient should repeat the maneuver to determine if it is reproducible. Each patient should have a plan of treatment that has been worked out with the physician. This will typically call for immediate use of rapidly acting bronchodilator medication delivered as an aerosol. The plan should contain instructions on the use of corticosteroids and notification of the patient's physician. An example of a treatment plan is seen in Figure 11. It should be remembered that a treatment plan must be individualized for each patient.

The physician's knowledge of the patient's history will prove invaluable at this time. Patients who have required hospitalization and especially those who have required respirator support for treatment of asthmatic attacks in the past will be advised not to delay treatment decisions. This patient group may require emergency room treatment as will patients with severe attacks who do not rapidly increase their peak flows with bronchodilator medication administered as directed (and not overused).

In treatment of bronchial asthma it is necessary to be aggressive early in treatment of severe attacks including the possible use of an emergency room. With early recognition of a severe attack and aggressive treatment at its onset fatal or near-fatal episodes can be avoided.

Francis V. Adams, M.D.
Pulmonary Medicine

Treatment Program for:
Jane Doe

Treatment
_____

Peak Flow Meter: Record your peak flow twice a day. Perform 3 efforts and take the best one. Your predicted normal is 400 l/min.

Asthma Treatment Plan: If your peak flow drops to 300 l/min: increase your bronchodilator spray to every 6 hours on a regular basis. Increase your steroid spray by doubling the number of sprays per day. If you have been using 4 puffs twice a day, increase to 8 puffs twice a day. If your peak flow decreases to 200 l/min: adjust the bronchodilator spray to every six hours and start Prednisone at 40mg a day. Speak to me as soon as possible. If your peak flow decreases to 100 l/min: use your bronchodilator spray immediately; start Prednisone 40mg and go to the nearest emergency room. Inform this office as soon as possible.

Please call if you have any questions regarding this treatment plan.

Figure 11. Sample of written treatment plan

In the patient group with severe attacks who respond promptly to treatment, the patient's treatment plan may often be continued in the home. With severe attacks this will most certainly require corticosteroids. Communication with the physician is essential and will be more accurate with serial peak flow measurements. Increasing airflows will confirm the effectiveness of treatment and can be used to adjust medication dosage and frequency of administration.

Following a severe attack that has been successfully treated it is important for the physician and patient to reassess maintenance medication and the treatment plan. The diary of peak flows will be extremely helpful since it may identify a downward trend that began before a severe attack was recognized. Emphasis on earlier recognition may prove helpful in avoiding future attacks.

With each significant attack the physician will look for a "trigger" mechanism that might be prevented in the future. An example would be raking moldy leaves or dusting without a facemask. Avoiding allergens will be stressed in sensitive patients who suffer serious attacks on exposure to these substances. Often the trigger for an asthmatic attack is the common cold. Although this infection cannot be prevented, the patient should be alerted to the possible adverse effects that might result and be prepared to institute the treatment plan.

In many instances the trigger for a severe asthmatic attack cannot be identified. If attacks are frequent, a review of the medical evaluation should be made. Additional allergy tests may be indicated and another careful examination of the home and work environment made. The patient's administration of medication should also be examined and the maintenance medication program reviewed.

What If Avoidance Doesn't Work?

Despite measures to avoid asthma triggers, the patient may still experience asthmatic attacks. These attacks may be frequent and severe and at times require hospitalization. In a small number of patients these attacks may prove fatal. In the next chapter, the asthma medications that are included in a treatment plan will be discussed.

The Asthma Medications

AS noted in chapter 3 an asthma treatment plan will include medication that the physician prescribes after the diagnosis has been made. In this chapter the different types of asthma medications and the methods used for their administration will be discussed. Asthma medication may be roughly divided into two groups. The first group includes medications that reverse the tightness or constriction in the bronchial tubes. These medications are called bronchodilators. The second group of medication is aimed at preventing future attacks. These medications are often called anti-inflammatory since they reverse the red, swollen appearance of the inside of the bronchial tubes. The anti-inflammatory medications are *not* used to treat a sudden asthmatic attack.

Bronchodilator Drugs

Beta-Agonists

Since asthma is characterized by narrowing of bronchial tubes caused by tightening of bronchial wall muscle, treatment has traditionally focused on reversing this process, which is called bronchodilatation. The medications that produce this effect are bronchodilators. At this time the most effective bronchodilators are the B_2-adrenergic agonists. These drugs are all derivatives of epinephrine which has effects on both the heart (termed beta-1) and lung (beta-2). Epinephrine is an important hormone produced in the body by the adrenal gland but has been synthesized in the laboratory. The B_2-adrenergic agonists have been developed to be "selective" stimulants of lung structures avoiding unwanted effects on the heart and blood vessels such as high blood pressure and palpitations. Their effects are produced through nerve endings called receptors located within the lungs. One such B_2-receptor is located in the muscle layer that surrounds the bronchial tube. With the administration of these agents and stimulation of the receptor the bronchial wall muscle relaxes producing bronchodilatation.

Are the B_2-Agonists Too Effective?

This potent and effective group of medications is now the subject of much debate. In the past these agents were often regarded as the only medication necessary for the treatment of asthma. Research has now shown that the B_2-adrenergic agonists do not have anti-inflammatory effects nor do they affect bronchial hyperresponsiveness. In view of these facts it has become increasingly clear that they cannot be relied on for the entire treatment of more than mild asthma.

It is also clear that despite their extreme effectiveness as bronchodilators their overuse may be a problem. Unfortunately, overuse of the B_2-agonists is extremely common. Statistics have shown a connection with overuse of one of the B-adrenergic agonists, fenoterol, and fatal asthma. It is not completely clear, however, whether this connection is due to a direct effect of over administration of this drug or whether it is simply due to the fact that a more severe group of asthmatics were using it. Several researchers have argued that these severe patients may suffer fatal attacks whether they overuse these agents or not.

Because of the rapid effect of alleviating asthma that is achieved by the B-agonists, patients tend to favor this group of medications over the slower-acting asthma drugs. It is not unusual to find that an asthmatic has stopped using other medications because "they didn't work like my other spray." In this way, patients will often fall into a pattern of overuse of this group of medications. It should be stressed that the use of the short-acting B_2-agonists should be on an "as needed" basis whenever possible. This alone identifies a patient who is under good control and has mild asthma. It should also be stressed that other asthma medications can be just as effective in controlling asthma if used properly.

Another area of controversy concerning the B_2-adrenergic agonists is that they are "too effective" and permit patients to expose themselves to unwanted and potentially harmful irritants. A 28-year-old woman with asthma and severe allergy to cat dander has been under my care for several years. On several office visits for flare-ups of her asthma she mentioned she had recently visited the homes of friends who had cats because she "knew my spray would help me." In fact she described many visits that ended with her making a "quick exit" even with the use of her B_2-agonist. Each visit would result in overuse of her spray. After discussing the dangers of overuse and the fact that the "late phase" of her attacks might explain why she was not doing well for days after her visits, the patient no longer places herself at unnecessary risk. Unfortunately, many patients continue to do so.

Long-Term Effects of B_2-Agonists

One of the most frequent questions that I am asked is whether there are any long-term effects of this group of medications. There is some evidence that use of B-adrenergic agonists may result in an increase in bronchial irritability when they are stopped, producing more asthma. This phenomenon does not appear to be significant when these agents are used as prescribed but may occur with overuse. If increased irritability does occur, it does not appear to be prolonged.

Another common question is whether the effect of the B_2-agonist "wears off" over time. This concern may lead to *underuse* of an important asthma medication. The great majority of studies of long-term use have not demonstrated that these agents lose their effectiveness. This phenomenon should not occur if the daily dosage is within the limits the physician prescribes but has been seen with overuse. It should be emphasized that the B-adrenergic agonists are safe and effective bronchodilators when used as directed by the physician. Both of the adverse effects noted above result from patients exceeding the prescribed dosage.

Specific Drugs: Old and New

The B-agonists were developed in the 1940s with isoproterenol the first of the class. Like epinephrine (adrenaline) this agent has both beta-1 and beta-2 effects. Isoetharine was one of the first "selective" B_2-adrenergic agonists introduced in the United States and it was followed by metaproterenol. With the development of selective B_2-adrenergic agonists there is no place for the use of non-selective agents that have significant stimulatory effects on the heart and circulation. Further research has produced more potent and longer-acting selective agents.

For the Acute Asthmatic Attack: Short-Acting Agent

Several selective B_2-adrenergic agonists are available for use. These agents are available as aerosol sprays delivered by metered-dose inhalers (MDIs), aerosol solution to be delivered by nebulization, dry powders for inhalation (DPI), short- and long-acting tablets and as syrups flavored for children. In the acute asthmatic attack the treatment of choice for prompt relief of symptoms is the administration of a short-acting B_2-adrenergic agonist. B_2-adrenergic agonists (albuterol, metaproterenol, pirbuterol, terbutaline, fenoterol, and bitolterol) have a rapid onset of action (within minutes) with a duration of action of four to six hours. The recommended dosage is two puffs every six hours as needed. These medications differ in potency as well as how fast they begin to work and when their peak effect is reached. There are also differences in how long the effect of the drug lasts. Fenoterol has never been made available in the United States. Its extremely rapid onset of action may have contributed to its overuse and it has been implicated in cases of fatal asthma in New Zealand. Table 1 lists the B_2-agonists by generic and brand name as well as the types of preparations that are available.

Long-Acting B_2-Agonists

Longer-acting B-adrenergic agonists (salmeterol, formoterol) delivered by metered-dose inhaler have been developed with a duration of action of up to twelve hours. These agents represent an exciting advance in the treatment of bronchial asthma and should be used for maintenance therapy.

Salmeterol

Salmeterol is currently available in the United States. The recommended dosage is two puffs every twelve hours administered on a regular basis. When compared to albuterol, salmeterol is more potent and more selective. Studies that have compared these two agents have documented that the salmeterol-treated patients have more sustained improvement in their lung function and fewer flare-ups of their asthma. In these studies the salmeterol patients also had fewer nocturnal attacks and awoke with better peak flows.

The longer-acting B-agonists appear to provide the patient with a more sustained control over their asthmatic symptoms, particularly patients with frequent nocturnal attacks. In addition, the twice-a-day administration provides greater convenience for the patient. Of note, however, the onset of action of the long-acting B-agonists is thirty to forty-five minutes. In view of this delayed onset the long-acting B-agonists should not be used for relief of an acute asthmatic attack.

After the introduction of salmeterol in the United States several deaths were reported in patients who suffered sudden asthmatic attacks and were not aware of the delayed onset of action of this drug. These patients

TABLE 1.   THE B-ADRENERGIC AGONISTS

Drug Name	Brand Name	Preparations	Comments
Albuterol	Proventil, Ventolin	MDI, DPI, Tablet, nebulizer, syrup	Selective, short to medium duration
Bitolterol	Tornalate	MDI, nebulizer	Selective
Isoetharine	Bronkosol, Bronkometer	MDI, nebulizer	Selective, short duration
Fenoterol	Berotec	MDI	Selective, not available in USA
Metaproterenol	Alupent, Metaprel	MDI, nebulizer, tablet, syrup	Less selective
Pirbuterol	Maxair	MDI, Autohaler	Selective
Salmeterol	Serevent	MDI	Selective, long duration
Terbutaline	Brethaire, Brethine, Bricanyl	MDI, injection,tablets	Selective, DPI available in Europe

should have been instructed to use a short-acting agent for their acute attacks. Some patients were not informed that both the short- and long-acting agents could be used together. Salmeterol represents a significant advance in the treatment of bronchial asthma. This drug should only be used for maintenance therapy, however, and does not have a role in the treatment of a sudden asthma attack.

Both the short- and long-acting agents administered before exercise are capable of preventing exercise-induced asthma (EIA). Salmeterol has been compared to albuterol in patients with exercise-induced asthma and appears to have an advantage. The salmeterol-treated patients had more sustained protection against EIA.

How Should the B-Adrenergic Agonist Be Given?

In an acute attack the fastest means of getting this medication to the bronchial tubes is by inhalation. This can be achieved in minutes by inhaling medicated spray administered by a metered-dose inhaler or powder delivered by a simple hand-held device. A medicated mist generated by a nebulizer can also be used for inhalation.

What Is an Asthma Aerosol?

An asthma aerosol is a mixture of a liquid medication suspended in a gas that can be inhaled. Aerosols differ in the size of the spray or mist particles that are inhaled. Particle size is important since large particles are not likely to reach the bronchial tubes and may land in the mouth or throat. Examples of asthma aerosols are sprays from metered-dose inhalers (MDIs) and nebulizers. The goal of aerosol therapy is inhalation of active medication with penetration into the bronchial tubes.

Metered-Dose Inhalers

Metered-dose inhalers contain medication in aerosol form. These devices were first introduced in 1956 and have become widely used for asthma and rhinitis. MDIs consist of a canister of medication and an actuator with

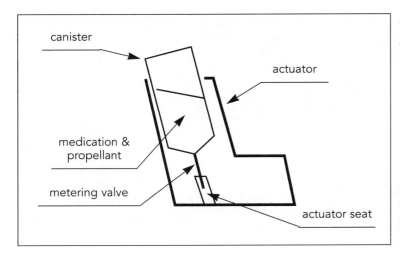

Figure 12. (left) Diagram of metered-dose inhaler

Figure 13. (below) Diagram of metered-dose inhaler with spacer

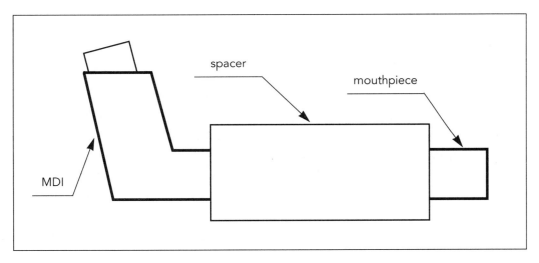

a mouthpiece. The actuator is the outer shell in which the canister "sits." In the canister, medication is suspended in a mixture of a liquid propellant gas and preservatives. The current propellant used in MDIs is a mixture of freon gases called chlorofluorocarbons.

When the canister is pressed into the actuator, the mixture of medication and propellant passes through a valve. The release of the contents under pressure transforms the liquid mixture into a spray that can be inhaled. In Figure 12 a metered-dose inhaler is diagramed. Figure 13 shows a metered-dose inhaler with a device known as a "spacer" attached.

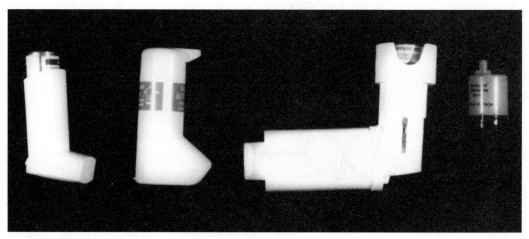

Figure 14.
Examples of MDIs and DPI (far right)

The metered-dose inhaler is the most common means of administration of the B-adrenergic agonists. It is a compact and portable device which dispenses a certain amount of medication rapidly. Coordination between hand activation of the MDI and breathing must exist for medication to be properly delivered. Metered-dose inhalers come in many shapes and sizes. Figure 14 shows several MDIs that are commonly used.

Although the metered-dose inhaler is in general a safe device it should be noted that a small number of patients may have adverse reactions to the propellants. This reaction may produce a worsening of asthma symptoms instead of the expected improvement after use of the MDI. Patients must also be careful to keep the mouthpiece of the metered-dose inhaler closed when not in use and free of foreign objects. Many patients have inadvertently aspirated foreign objects such as coins which slipped into the open mouthpiece and were then inhaled. MDIs are frequently kept in a pocket or purse where such foreign objects are usually found so that it is best to carefully check the MDI before its use.

A 32-year-old man under my care for bronchial asthma called me in distress one night stating that "something went wrong when I sprayed." He had been in the habit of keeping his uncovered MDI in his pocket and while shopping had placed loose change in the same pocket. After dinner he had used his MDI and felt "something go in." An x-ray in the emergency room showed a dime lodged in his windpipe. A procedure called bronchoscopy was required to remove it. The patient was released the next day with a MDI that he had carefully capped.

Nebulizers

A nebulizer may also be used to rapidly deliver aerosol medication containing B-adrenergic agonists. This device, which is commonly used in an emergency room setting, is basically a simple system that allows rapidly flowing air or oxygen to be bubbled through a solution containing the drug. This system produces a vapor that the patient inhales. Nebulizers differ in terms of the size of mist particles they produce. Of note, the nebulizer does not require coordination between hand and breathing necessary for MDI use.

Nebulizer delivery of a B-agonist is preferred in emergency settings due to the greater quantity of drug that can be delivered. This has been

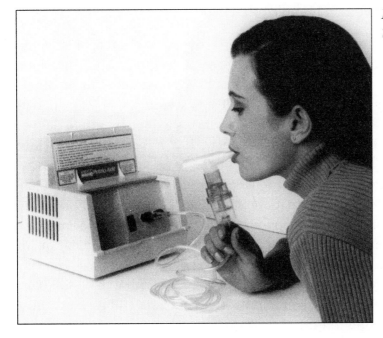

Figure 15.
Using a nebulizer

estimated to be approximately from four to ten times the amount of medication delivered by two puffs from a metered-dose inhaler. The greater quantity of drug delivered by the nebulizer method may also result in greater side effects (tremors, rapid heart beat, muscle cramps, nervousness) than those noted after metered-dose inhalation. In an emergency setting the beneficial effect of opening the bronchial tubes usually outweighs any adverse side effects.

Nebulizers may be obtained for the home but this should not be necessary for most asthma patients. In view of the adverse effects and increased dosage noted above, a home nebulizer should only be prescribed for the most severely afflicted patients with asthma that cannot be controlled with metered-dose sprays or powder. These devices are much more expensive and cumbersome than MDIs, although portable units are available. In Figure 15 a patient is shown using a nebulizer.

One advantage of the nebulizer may be its ability to combine more than one drug in solution given as one treatment. It should be noted, however, that metered-dose inhalers with more than one medication are likely to be available soon.

Metered-Dose Inhaler Versus Nebulizer Delivery

A number of studies have compared the effectiveness of a B-agonist delivered by a metered-dose inhaler with a spacer attachment and the same drug delivered by a nebulizer. These studies have shown little or no difference in effectiveness between the two delivery systems. One explanation is that with a metered-dose spray the patient takes a deep breath to deliver medication to the bronchial tubes while with a nebulizer the patient breathes normally. The deep breath may actually be advantageous to the delivery of medication to smaller bronchial tubes. During a severe attack, however, it may be difficult for patients to actively inhale deeply enough. While routine use of a nebulizer for stable asthma should be discouraged, there remains a definite place for nebulizer-delivery of medication in patients with severe disease and in an emergency.

Nebulizers also require more maintenance and cleaning than do MDIs. There is a greater risk of contamination with nebulizers and patients must follow a proper cleaning routine.

Proper Technique for MDI Use: Open Mouth

Proper technique in the use of a metered-dose inhaler is essential to the effectiveness of the B-adrenergic agonist. It is estimated that only 10 to 14 percent of the medication released reaches the smaller, more peripheral airways of the lung. If the drug is not administered correctly symptoms will not be relieved, often leading to overuse.

Two methods of inhaling medication are commonly used. The preferred is the open-mouth technique since it has the potential to almost double the amount of medication delivered to the bronchial tubes. In this technique the MDI is held about an inch in front of the open mouth. It is best to practice with a mirror at home after being instructed in the doctor's office.

Before activating the spray first determine the amount of pressure needed by "test-firing" into the room. You may hold the MDI with both hands if necessary. Before activating the spray empty your lungs by exhaling. When you feel the need to inhale, activate the spray so that the medication will be maximally inhaled. Inhale slowly over three to five seconds, then hold your breath, if possible, by counting to five before exhaling again. Do not repeat the second spray in "rapid fire sequence." Allow at least a minute between sprays. Too often patients will "puff-puff" in a few seconds and then wonder why they have to use their inhalers again "so soon." Proper technique is essential for medication to reach the small airways of the lung. Figure 16 shows the proper technique used in the open-mouth method.

The alternative is the closed-mouth method, which most pharmaceutical package-insert instructions suggest. The patient performs the same maneuver but with the lips closed tightly around the mouthpiece. This technique is pictured in Figure 17. Although individual patients may find this effective, studies of the amount delivered have documented better delivery with the open-mouth method.

Always check the expiration date on the side of the removable metal canister and discard any expired medication. It is best to determine how many puffs are available by the number you have used (keep a record if necessary) or by the date obtained. Mark your calendar when you purchase your inhaler. Most MDIs contain 200 to 240 sprays and from your

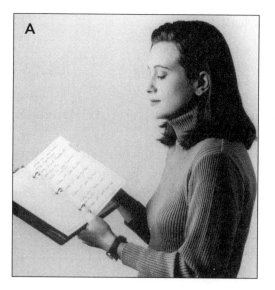
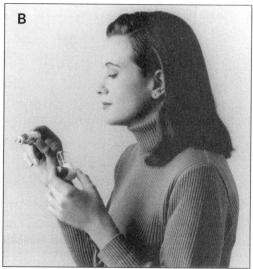

Figure 16.
Open Mouth Technique for MDI:
A (above left) First check your calender for date of purchase . . .
B (above right) Also check date of expiration on canister
C (below left) Shake MDI vigorously!
D (below right) Position MDI about an inch in front of open mouth

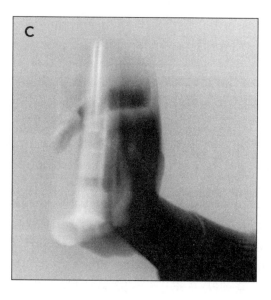
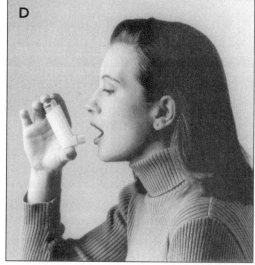

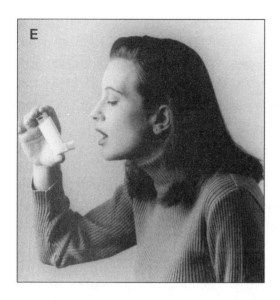

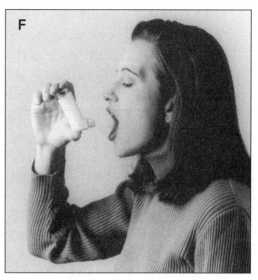

Figure 16. (continued)

E (above left) Let all the air out of your lungs (exhale)

F (above right) Spray and begin a slow, deep full breath (inhale)

G (below left) Hold your breath for 5–10 seconds (if possible)

H (below right) Exhale and relax: Wait 30–60 seconds and then
repeat steps C–H

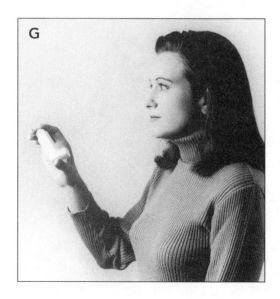

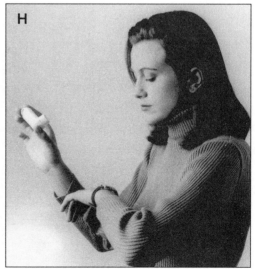

pattern of use it should be easy to calculate how long a spray will last. A test using a glass of water to determine if the metal canister will float (empty) or sink to the bottom (full) is less accurate than an actual record. Never assume medication is present by the "feel" of the weight of the MDI. Propellants and preservatives are used in MDIs and may give you the false impression that some medication remains.

Common Mistakes

Large studies have documented the difficulty that patients experience with metered-dose inhalers. It has been estimated that more than 50 percent of patients use improper technique with the most common mistake being the "firing" of the medication after inhalation begins. Poor coordination may not improve with repeated instruction. Additional common mistakes include failing to remove the cap and holding the spray upside down. Patients should be encouraged to have the physician observe their technique with the metered-dose inhaler. Videotapes of the proper technique are available and may be obtained from the physician.

Figure 17.
Closed mouth
technique for MDI use

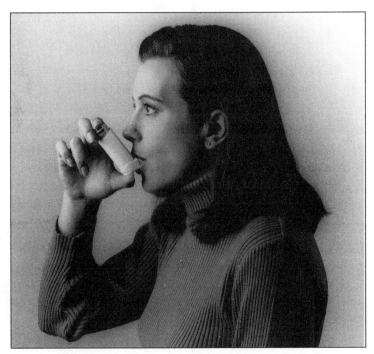

About 70 percent of the medication discharged on activation of the MDI is deposited in the mouth and throat and never reaches the bronchial tubes. Approximately 15 percent remains in the mouthpiece of the MDI and 10–25 percent actually reaches the bronchial airways. Any method that increases deposition of medication into the bronchi is advantageous to the control and treatment of asthma. For treatment to be successful, the coordination between activation of the MDI and inhalation must be fairly precise.

The Propellants

Metered-dose inhalers are currently pressurized by Freon propellants. These chloroflurocarbons (CFCs) are known to have an adverse effect on the environment by destroying the atmospheric ozone layer. Sweden has banned the manufacture of Freon-pressurized MDIs and many countries are likely to widen the ban by 1995. In the United States, CFC-pressurized aerosol devices are to be banned by the year 2000. It is likely, however, that a medical exemption for metered-dose inhalers will be added to this legislation. Substitutes for Freon that do not affect the ozone layer, such as HFC 134a, are currently undergoing testing and may be in use in the next two years.

Breath-Activated Inhaler

In view of the difficulty some patients have coordinating metered-dose inhalers, great interest has been devoted to the development of a breath-activated inhaler. Pirbuterol is available in this form (Maxair Autohaler) and additional breath-activated devices have been under development (see chapter 14). With the Autohaler the patient has to inhale forcefully, activating the mechanism that delivers the dosage of medication. Education in the use of a breath-activated device is also required but it appears patients achieve mastery of this device faster than with the MDI. In those patients who have good coordination with metered-dose inhalers, the breath-activated device does not appear to improve delivery of medication. In patients with poor coordination, however, the breath-activated inhaler will improve delivery of bronchodilator medication. A drawback of the Maxair Autohaler spray is the lack of an override button that would allow the patient to activate the spray if it malfunctions. In addition, patients with severe degrees of narrowing of the bronchial tubes may have difficulty activating the device.

Spacers

Patients who experience difficulty with metered-dose inhalers may benefit from the use of a spacer or extension tube. Spacers come in different sizes (large or small volume) and shapes. Figure 18 shows three spacer devices that are widely used.

The spacer in its simplest form consists of an attachment or holding chamber that fits over the mouthpiece of the MDI. Activation of the inhaler allows the medication to enter the attached chamber or "spacer" from which the patient then inhales. Use of this device often improves the delivery of medication since it is more difficult for the patient to "lose the medication" by spraying before inhaling. The medication is "trapped" in the spacer for several seconds allowing the patient to inhale with less fear of "spraying and inhaling at the wrong time."

Studies of various spacers have shown they reduce the amount of medication deposited in the mouth that never reaches the bronchial

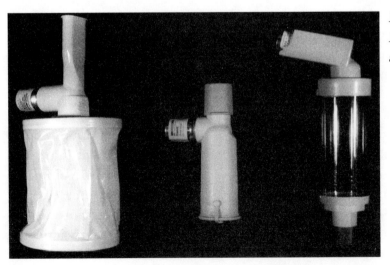

Figure 18.
Examples of
spacers

tubes. Even the simplest device has been shown to reduce by half the amount "lost" in the mouth. Although the amount of medication deposited in the mouth may be reduced by even the simplest spacer, it appears that the larger volume spacers actually increase the amount of medication that reaches the lungs. Examples of large-volume spacers are InspirEase, InhalAid, and Nebuhaler. InspirEase consists of a collapsible bag and a valve that can signal the patient when inhaling too fast. Aerochamber is a medium-sized spacer with a mouthpiece and one-way valve that can also signal if the patient is inhaling too fast. It is also available with a facemask for small children and adults (Figure 19). OptiHaler is an extremely compact spacer that easily incorporates the MDI in its design. Table 2 is a partial list of currently used spacers.

Patients with poor technique with a metered-dose inhaler may also experience difficulty with a large-volume spacer. As with the MDI it is important not to "fire" the medication after the start of a breath. Breathe in slowly to full inspiration. Some patients have been reluctant to "carry around" the larger spacers and feel they are cumbersome.

Advantages of a Spacer

Spacers may offer several other advantages with metered-dose inhalers. The total body absorption of inhaled medication is greatly influ-

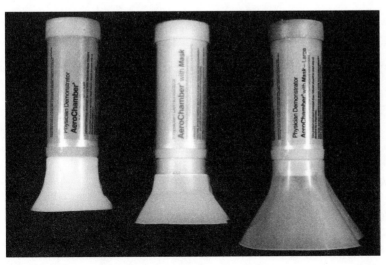

Figure 19.
Spacer with mask
attached in
different sizes

enced by the amount deposited in the mouth. This material makes up the highest proportion of medication that is absorbed. By reducing the amount lost in the mouth, spacers reduce total body absorption and may therefore reduce possible total body side effects. With the B-agonists, this may mean reduced nervousness or shakiness after use. This benefit may be advantageous in high doses of inhaled corticosteroids, reducing the chances of steroid side effects on the whole body. Spacers have also been shown to reduce the risk of yeast infection (candidiasis) that may occur with the inhaled corticosteroids.

Another advantage of a large-volume spacer is that in those patients requiring large numbers of puffs of medication, as in high-dose inhaled corticosteroids, the spacer allows the patient to inhale two puffs of medication for each inhalation, thus reducing the time the patient must spend inhaling large doses of medication.

Children and Spacers

In children, spacers may be extremely helpful in delivering medication. Children as young as three years of age who would not otherwise by able to use a MDI may benefit from the use of a spacer with a facemask (Aerochamber). Studies of children with asthma that have compared the use of a metered-dose inhaler with a spacer with mask and a nebulizer have found no difference in safety or effectiveness.

TABLE 2.   SPACER DEVICES*

Name	Size	Comments
Aerochamber	Medium Volume	Rigid, signals fast flow, available with mask for children
InspirEase	Large Volume	Collapsible bag, mouthpiece signals if inhaling too fast
Nebuhaler	Large Volume	Rigid, mouthpiece
OptiHaler	Small Volume	Compact, MDI canister may be carried in device

*This is a partial list of spacer devices and is not intended to be all-inclusive.

Dry Powder Inhalers

B$_2$-adrenergic agonists such as albuterol and salmeterol are also available in dry powder form for inhalation (salmeterol is not yet available in this form in the U.S.). Multidose dispensers are becoming increasingly available to assist patients in administering this powder with a minimum of preparation. Single-dose dry powder inhalers (DPI) are widely available. Figure 14 shows an example of a DPI. This form of medication may be particularly helpful with patients who have difficulty with MDIs since with the powder form the patient again performs a breath-activated inhalation after placing the lips tightly around the mouthpiece. In the same maneuver as performed with the MDI the patient first empties the lungs, then performs a maximal inhalation thus fully drawing in the powder and then holding the breath. With environmental concerns growing over the use of chlorofluorocarbon (CFC) propellants that destroy the ozone layer, the use of B-adrenergic agonists in powder form will increase. Patient acceptance of this form of medication has been slow primarily because of unfamiliarity as well as increased coughing and wheezing in addition to minor throat discomfort. However, the latter may also occur with the spray form as well as minor changes in voice noted by a few patients.

Patients with arthritis or neurologic diseases such as Parkinson's disease may experience difficulty loading the powder capsule into their inhaler. This problem will be eased by wider distribution of multiple-dose powder inhalers, currently available in Europe. Another possible drawback of powder inhalers is that the amount of medication the patient receives varies with the force of inhalation. Patients who can inhale more forcefully may receive a lot more medication. Another consideration with dry powder inhalers is the adverse effect of high humidity conditions on their function.

Dry powder inhalers are clearly not as versatile as metered-dose inhalers. Metered-dose inhalers have now been used with patients who are breathing with the assistance of a respirator. The MDI may be fitted with a special adapter that allows medication to be inhaled through the respirator system. For this and other reasons, it is clear that the MDI will remain in widespread use for treatment of bronchial asthma.

Oral Forms of B$_2$-Agonists

The B-adrenergic agonists available in tablet or elixir form are not for emergency use since they have slow onsets of action (up to one hour). Albuterol, terbutaline, and metaproterenol are available as oral medications. Since they are absorbed into the bloodstream in greater quantity than the inhaled form, there are greater chances of side effects. These include tremors, muscle cramps, nervousness, insomnia, and palpitations. The long-acting oral preparations of albuterol have proved useful for patients with nocturnal asthma although the long-acting aerosol sprays that have become available also have been effective in this setting. Those patients who have difficulty using a metered-dose inhaler may benefit from the oral preparations.

Another potential advantage of oral preparations is that the medication carried in the blood may reach small bronchial tubes that may not have been reached by inhalation. These small airways are often inflamed and swollen in moderate and severe asthma and receive only a relatively small percentage of the medication inhaled. In addition, there may be thick mucus "plugs" that block the air passages. Aerosol medication may therefore be primarily distributed to the larger, more open passages which receive greater airflow on inhalation. It is conceivable, however, that medication deposited in these larger passages may be absorbed into blood vessels and reach the blood circulation, thereby eventually reaching the smaller airways.

In the asthmatic patient who does not appear to respond fully to aerosol medication, trial with an oral preparation is indicated. Peak flows or spirometry may be performed after a suitable trial of one to two weeks. If flow rates have increased and symptoms have diminished then the oral preparation of the B$_2$-adrenergic agonist may be used in conjunction with the aerosol. A drawback to this approach will be the greater likelihood of adverse effects from the increased absorption of the B-agonist. Of note, however, is that tolerance to these effects often develops after several days of use. Unfortunately, the elderly population with asthma may be adversely affected more than younger patients. Tremors may be especially severe in older patients. These patients are also more likely to have preexisting cardiac conditions that may increase the risk of adverse effects such as rapid or irregular heart rhythms.

Should Epinephrine Ever Be Used?

The use of epinephrine by injection for the treatment of asthma dates to as early as 1903. An aerosol form was developed around 1910. For many decades epinephrine was the only available medication for the treatment of bronchial asthma. Its use in the emergency setting has certainly saved countless numbers of lives.

In view of the fact that epinephrine is a non-selective agent that has potent effects on the heart and circulation, its use for treating bronchial asthma has declined. In elderly patients in particular, administration of epinephrine may result in increases in blood pressure and heart rate. These effects may contribute to the development of stroke and heart attack. For these reasons, emergency room treatment of bronchial asthma usually consists of the administration of a selective B-adrenergic agonist by nebulization.

For Anaphylaxis

Epinephrine is still an important medication for treating severe allergic reactions. It is the treatment of choice for a severe reaction known as anaphylaxis, a severe total body allergic reaction that may lead to collapse or shock. One example would be the severe reaction to a bee sting in a sensitive individual. Injectable preparations of epinephrine that automatically inject a pre-measured dose are available by prescription for highly allergic patients.

Over-the-Counter Medication

Over-the-counter nonprescription preparations of aerosol epinephrine should be avoided. These preparations are extremely weak and short acting with effects that may last only a few minutes and therefore are commonly abused. With the far more effective treatment available for bronchial asthma I feel these agents would best be withdrawn since they may actually deter patients from seeking appropriate and necessary medical attention.

Theophylline

Theophylline has been used for treating bronchial asthma for nearly sixty years but is a weaker bronchodilator than the B-adrenergic agonists. Although widely used as a bronchodilator the mechanism of its action is unclear. The most recent theories suggest an anti-inflammatory effect that is supported by the inhibition of the late phase response. Due to the controversy over its mode of action, theophylline has fallen out of favor and is no longer regarded as a first-line asthma medication comparable to the B_2-adrenergic agonists. As more data is obtained that firmly establishes theophylline as an anti-inflammatory agent it is likely to be regarded again as a first-line agent.

At this time theophylline may still prove useful as a second-line drug. Patients with intolerance to B-agonist side effects may find they are better able to tolerate theophylline. Its availability as an oral medication in a sustained time-release form may be preferred by some patients. Dosing is usually on a twice-a-day basis with some patients able to achieve satisfactory results from once-a-day administration. This once-a-day dose is best given in the evening and may prove extremely helpful in treating nocturnal asthma.

Sustained-Release Preparations

Large numbers of sustained-release theophylline preparations are available by prescription, but they may vary in their rate of release of medication into the bloodstream. Once a certain preparation is prescribed, adjustment of the dosage will require follow-up and blood testing. After the proper dosage is established it is advisable not to substitute one preparation for another since the substitute may not achieve the same results. There is little use for short-acting theophylline preparations since they must be given several times a day.

Intravenous Form: Aminophylline

An intravenous form of theophylline known as aminophylline is available for emergencies. In view of the faster onset of action of the B_2-adrenergic agonists intravenous aminophylline would also not be considered a first-line treatment in an emergency room. Although there is some controversy concerning its effectiveness in emergencies, aminophylline as a second-line agent has been established.

Obtaining a Therapeutic Level

One drawback to theophylline is that a certain amount must be present to achieve an effect. This has been termed a therapeutic level (10–20 mg of the drug per liter of blood). Some patients, however, may benefit from lower levels. To achieve the therapeutic level a certain dosage must be administered. Dosing is based on patient body weight and when given by mouth may require several adjustments based on blood test results before achieving a patient's daily maintenance dose. When theophylline is given by mouth an effect may be achieved in approximately one hour but it may require two to three days to achieve the desired maintenance level. With intravenous administration of aminophylline a "loading dose" is usually given over thirty minutes followed by a constant infusion. Blood levels are again required to adjust the intravenous drip. Compared to the rapidly acting B-agonists, theophylline is both weaker and slower in producing bronchodilatation. Of note, however, when theophylline is given at the same time that the patient is receiving the B-agonist, the effect of the two drugs together may be greater than when given alone.

Adverse Effects of Theophylline

Besides the above considerations, theophylline may have significant side effects, often related to high blood levels, but some patients may experience adverse effects on small dosages, including stomach and bowel upset, rapid or irregular heart beat, insomnia, nervousness, urinary frequency, and headache. Some of these effects may be prevented or reduced by avoiding caffeine, which is structurally similar to theophylline, which explains why coffee has often been noted to relieve asthma. Patients should be advised to avoid or reduce caffeine in their diets while receiving theophylline.

Children and Theophylline

One disturbing but controversial side effect has been noted in children. A possible adverse effect on learning and behavior has been raised by some studies. There are conflicting results with additional studies that have not demonstrated these effects. At this time, theophylline should be used with caution in young children. Careful monitoring for changes in behavior patterns and learning must be performed.

Overdosage

In excessive or toxic dosages, theophylline may cause nausea, vomiting, irregular heart rhythms, and seizures. Theophylline should never be used without direction and supervision from the physician. Fatalities have been reported in asthmatics who have overused over-the-counter asthma medications that contain theophylline. These OTC preparations should be withdrawn to avoid toxic reactions.

Drugs that Interact with Theophylline

Another important consideration when patients receive theophylline is the potential for drug interaction. This interaction may result in higher blood levels or toxicity from theophylline. One major group of drugs that can interact with theophylline are certain antibiotics, including erythromycin, clarithromycin, ciprofloxacin, and olfloxacin. In addition, a widely prescribed stomach medication, cimetadine (Tagamet), may also interact with theophylline. Fortunately, many other antibiotics and stomach medications are compatible with theophylline. In instances where one of the drugs that may interact with theophylline must be given, a reduction in the theophylline dosage may be made in order to avoid toxicity. A simple rule is to cut in half the total daily dose whenever receiving one of the above medications. It is vital to monitor blood levels in that situation.

Factors that Affect Theophylline Breakdown

Other factors may contribute to slower breakdown or clearance of theophylline, such as age, liver disease, and heart disease. Elderly patients have been found to clear theophylline more slowly. Patients with diseases of the liver as well as those with congestive heart failure have also been found to have slower metabolism of theophylline. In these groups, lower dosages of theophylline should be given.

Some drugs may accelerate clearance of theophylline from the body. Cigarette and marijuana smokers are often found to clear theophylline more rapidly than nonsmokers and may need their dosages increased. Two medications used for epilepsy, phenytoin (Dilantin) and phenobarbital may also increase breakdown of theophylline.

Anticholinergic Drugs

For thousands of years it has been observed that anticholinergic drugs had beneficial effects on many patients with respiratory diseases. In fact, many ancient herbal preparations have been found to include atropine (from leaves of the *Atropa belladonna* plant) and stramonium (from the plant *Datura stramonium*). Stramonium cigarettes were commonly smoked in the late nineteenth century for relief of asthma.

Atropine

Physicians have long used atropine for patients with breathing disorders including asthma. Until recently, however, use of atropine and similar agents has been limited by the total body absorption of these medications, short duration of action and the side effects they produce. One disturbing adverse effect is drying of secretions in the respiratory tract. In bronchial asthma this effect may result in increased "plugging" of the bronchial tubes, thereby worsening the attack. Other adverse effects include difficulty with urination (retention), visual changes including blurring of vision and worsening of narrow-angle glaucoma, mental changes including agitation, and dry mouth. It is also important to note that the benefit of these drugs in bronchial asthma was mild and that they were regarded as weak bronchodilators.

Ipratropium Bromide

The recent introduction of an anticholinergic drug, ipratropium bromide, that was not absorbed to any degree into the total body circulation has permitted the use of this agent in diseases characterized by bronchoconstriction. Due to the extremely small amount of absorption of this drug, no drying effect on bronchial mucus has been noted. Ipratropium bromide (Atrovent) is available as an aerosol medication for metered-dose inhalers and in solution for nebulization. The recommended MDI dosage is two puffs every six hours. It should be noted that ipratropium bromide has a slow onset of action that may not peak for sixty minutes. The nebulizer solution may be combined with solutions of the B-adrenergic agonists.

How Anticholinergic Agents Work

The action of the anticholinergic agent is believed to be primarily on the tone of the bronchial wall muscle. This muscle tone is thought to be controlled in part by the vagus nerve, a component of the nervous pathway called the cholinergic nervous system. Cholinergic receptors coexist in bronchial wall muscle with the adrenergic receptors. When the cholinergic receptor is stimulated the activity of the vagus nerve is reduced, resulting in relaxation of the bronchial muscle and bronchodilatation.

A Better Drug for Emphysema

In bronchial asthma the role of the cholinergic system is minor and therefore the effect of anticholinergic drugs is weak compared to B-adrenergic agonists. The anticholinergic agents have no anti-inflammatory effects and no effect on the late phase of bronchial asthma or on bronchial hyperresponsiveness. However, anticholinergic agents are of greater value for patients with emphysema and chronic bronchitis where it is clear that the vagal cholinergic tone plays a greater role in bronchoconstriction. Those patients with bronchial asthma who have components of emphysema and chronic bronchitis from cigarette abuse or recurrent infection may be good subjects for a trial of ipratropium bromide, but this trial should only occur after primary use of B_2-adrenergic agonists.

Adverse Effects

Adverse effects of ipratropium bromide are few. Small numbers of patients have noted a bitter taste and headache. Rare reports of increased wheezing after use of the nebulizer solution have been noted. Patients with narrow-angle glaucoma and enlargement of the prostate gland should avoid it.

When to Use

Once patients have had an adequate trial of B_2-adrenergic agonists, those who remain symptomatic with evidence of airway obstruction should be considered candidates for trials of theophylline and/or the anticholinergics to increase bronchodilatation.

Anti-Inflammatory Drugs

Inhaled Corticosteroids

With greater emphasis being placed on the inflammatory nature of bronchial asthma, the anti-inflammatory agents have achieved greater importance in treatment. The most effective anti-inflammatory agents are corticosteroids, limited to oral or injectable forms until relatively recently when an inhalation form became available. The topically active inhaled steroids have radically changed and improved the treatment of bronchial asthma. Patients who would have previously been dependent on oral steroids with serious lifetime consequences have been able to be maintained on the spray with virtually no side effects. Those patients with milder forms of asthma but who overuse bronchodilator drugs have been able to decrease their consumption of these agents, reducing the adverse effects of these drugs and perhaps avoiding fatal attacks.

How They Work

Corticosteroids reduce inflammation in the bronchial tubes. Steroids prevent the late phase response and reduce bronchial hyperresponsiveness. The inhaled corticosteroids (beclomethasone dipropionate, triamcinolone acetonide, flunisolide, budesonide, fluticasone) are "topically active" and achieve their effect on the surface of the bronchial lining. Many of these same agents are used as creams or ointments for skin conditions. If you visualize the lining of the bronchial tube in asthma to be red and inflamed then the application of the steroid spray is not unlike applying a steroid cream to a skin rash. The results may be a dramatic reduction in inflammation and irritability.

It must be emphasized that for corticosteroids to be effective they must be administered regularly. Too often patients may abandon a steroid inhaler before it has a chance to work. Compared to the B-adrenergic agonists, corticosteroids do not have an immediate effect and cannot rapidly reduce symptoms. For this reason patients may stop this important medication before it has had an adequate trial. Remember that the primary purpose of corticosteroid sprays is prevention. If used correctly these agents may provide long-term control over asthma. Another major benefit of the regular use of inhaled corticosteroid sprays is the reduced need for B_2-agonists, which is extremely important in view of the detrimental effects noted from overusing B_2-adrenergic agents.

Specific Agents

Table 3 lists the inhaled corticosteroids, their brand names, and the forms that are available. Beclomethasone dipropionate, triamcinolone acetonide, and flunisolide are available in the United States. Budesonide, which has been used extensively in Europe and Canada, is available in the United States as a nasal spray and should be released soon for inhalation. Fluticasone has recently become available in the United States as a nasal spray and should be available for inhalation in the near future.

Dosage and Administration

These agents may be given in varying dosages depending on individual patients. A common starting dose would be 400 micrograms (ug) or eight puffs per day of one of the inhaled corticosteroids. Comparison of the three agents currently available in the United States has found a similar degree of effectiveness. The dose of the inhaled steroid may be given on a twice-a-day basis instead of the four times a day usually prescribed. This will often improve patient compliance and may even be adjusted to once a day for patients who are stable and liable to miss dosages. For adult patients with severe asthma dosages as high as twenty puffs a day (2.0 mg) may be used without evidence of total body absorption. In children, however, evidence of absorption has been noted with dosages over 400 ug per day.

'High-Dose' Sprays

In view of the large number of sprays needed on a daily basis, "high-dose" sprays have been made available with up to 250 ug per puff of corticosteroid. These inhalers allow patients with stable asthma to be maintained on as little as two puffs twice a day. Flunisolide is the only "high-dose" inhaler currently available in the United States.

Adverse Effects and How to Prevent Them

The primary side effect of inhaled corticosteroids is development of a yeast infection known as candidiasis in the mouth or throat. With large numbers of puffs from the "low-dose" inhaler or the use of the "high-dose" preparation, there is a greater risk of this infection. This is a local infection and the rare instances of its spreading outside the mouth have typically occurred in patients with lowered immunity who took no precautionary steps. Several preventive steps can be taken to avoid the infection, including rinsing the mouth after spraying. If unable to rinse the patient may simply drink, flushing residual medication away from the mouth and throat. Passage through the digestive tract leads to rapid breakdown of the drug but rinsing is still preferred. Another extremely helpful step in administering inhaled steroid aimed at reducing the risk of yeast infection is a spacer. This simple device improves delivery of the steroid to the lung as well as reducing the amount likely to be deposited in the mouth and throat. Triamcinolone acetonide (Azmacort) incorporates a spacer in its MDI. If candidiasis is discovered, treatment should be given promptly, consisting usually of an antifungal agent (nystatin, clortrimazole) prepared as a mouthwash or as a lozenge. It is rare that development of an oral yeast infection will recur and prompt discontinuation of inhaled steroids. In patients with recurrent yeast infection a switch to another anti-inflammatory agent such as cromolyn sodium or nedocromil would be indicated.

Another infrequent side effect of inhaled steroids is an effect on voice. This uncommon effect is usually noted as hoarseness and may be alleviated with a spacer and by temporary reduction in dosage. Patients who complain of changes in voice should have a careful examination of the vocal cords to ensure that there is no other explanation for the abnormality.

Are Inhaled Steroid Sprays Really Safe?

There is often great fear on the part of patients when the discussion of asthma medication turns to corticosteroids. This may explain why these agents are greatly underused. It is common to associate inhaled steroids with the side effects of oral or injected steroid drugs. Inhaled steroids are not absorbed in appreciable amounts into the bloodstream and total body and they are *not* the bodybuilding steroids that have received so much media attention. The minor and infrequent side effects noted above are usually not significant and rarely cause a patient to stop treatment. In adults large dosages are clearly as safe as low dosages. In children the normal dosages prescribed have not been found to produce significant side effects. Higher dosages in children may have effects on bone growth but usually can be avoided with the use of an alternative anti-inflammatory drug such as cromolyn sodium.

How Soon Should I See an Effect?

A reasonable trial of an inhaled corticosteroid will often require two to three weeks. At that point dosage may have to be adjusted to achieve a significant effect over an additional two to three weeks.

How Long Must I Remain on My Steroid Spray?

Long-term studies have determined that the benefits of inhaled topical corticosteroids are not maximized for periods approaching one year of use. There is clearly a slow onset of action and patients who abandon their medication at three months or less clearly are deprived of further benefits from continued use. "Can I be cured of my asthma by a steroid spray?" is a frequent question asked by patients. The answer is that a cure is unlikely and infrequent. Individual patients treated for at least one year with a steroid spray have been able to discontinue medication and remain well but long-term follow-up is lacking in these patients. It should be emphasized that bronchial asthma is usually a chronic disease and that treatment is often for life.

Do I Have to Use My B-Agonist Spray Before My Steroid Spray?

It has been a common and widespread practice to give a B-adrenergic agonist before the inhaled steroid spray. The reasoning has been to facilitate the entry and penetration of the steroid medication. In stable patients, however, it has been demonstrated that this is not necessary and patients may use their steroid spray alone and achieve equal delivery of medication. Patients who are wheezing or who note increased cough after their steroid spray may be helped by premedication with the B-agonist. If the two agents are used together it is important to allow five to ten minutes between them, enough time for the B-agonist to achieve significant bronchodilatation before the steroid is applied.

Systemic Corticosteroids

Before introduction of inhaled corticosteroids in the 1970s, these agents were limited to oral or injectable preparations that produced total body or systemic effects. Many patients with bronchial asthma became steroid

TABLE 3. INHALED CORTICOSTEROIDS

Drug	Brand Name	Strength ug/puff	Form	Comment
Beclomethasone dipropionate	Beclovent, Vanceril	42	MDI	High dose (250) (Becloforte) and DPI (Becotide, Becodisks) available in Canada, Europe
Budesonide	Pulmicort	50, 200, 400	MDI, DPI	Available in Canada, Europe
Flunisolide	Aerobid	250	MDI	Mint flavor form, Aerobid-M
Fluticasone propionate	Flixotide, Flovent	50, 100, 200	DPI, MDI	Available in Europe
Triamcinolone acetonide	Azmacort	100	MDI	Incorporates spacer device

dependent for life and developed serious side effects. Although inhaled corticosteroids have spared many patients this "life sentence" or allowed many to reduce their steroid dosages, systemic corticosteroids are still often required to treat acute and severe bronchial asthma.

When Should Systemic Steroids Be Used?

In patients with severe attacks who are already receiving bronchodilator and anti-inflammatory therapy a course of an oral steroid such as prednisone, prednisolone or methylprednisolone will be necessary. Those patients who require emergency room care and/or hospitalization will often require intravenous preparations of hydrocortisone (Solucortef) or methylprednisolone (Solumedrol). In treating severe asthma the most common error is to undertreat with smaller dosages of steroid than necessary. This error often arises from the concern for the development of adverse effects, although a short course of corticosteroids usually produces few side effects. If adverse effects do develop, they are usually transient and quickly resolve after the course of steroids is concluded.

Dosages of Oral Corticosteroids

A typical short course of oral steroid in the setting of a severe attack resistant to the patient's maintenance and contingent medications would start at a dosage of prednisone (or an equivalent dosage of methylprednisolone) of 40–60 mg a day. Patients with more severe disease with a history of requiring courses of oral steroid are more likely to require the higher dosage. Depending on the severity of the attack this dosage may be maintained from one to seven days before it is reduced and the total course may extend from approximately one to three weeks. This tapering is especially necessary for the longer courses to allow the adrenal gland to function normally.

Considering the Adrenal Gland

The adrenal gland produces the body's own supply of cortisone. When this gland recognizes that corticosteroid is present in the bloodstream in quantities greater than usual it stops its own production. This is called adrenal suppression and the state of inactivity is termed adrenal insufficiency. In this state, the absence of cortisone under stressful conditions may produce low blood pressure and shock. The tapering of steroid dosages, however, allows the gland to recover function. For extremely brief courses, however, tapering is not necessary.

In-Hospital Use of Steroids

Patients who are hospitalized with severe attacks are usually treated with intravenous methylprednisolone (Solumedrol) in dosages varying between 40 and 60 mg intravenously every six hours. This dosage is usually maintained for one to three days, then tapered with transfer to an oral corticosteroid. The taper of the oral steroid may extend another one to three weeks. With high doses of intravenous or oral corticosteroid being administered the addition of the inhaled steroid does not contribute significantly to treatment. Inhaled corticosteroids are not valuable in treating acute attacks and should be considered prophylactic medications. Therefore, they are usually introduced or restarted after the acute attack symptoms have greatly improved. Due to slow onset of action it is helpful to overlap the lower tapering dosages of the oral steroid and the inhaled form. A good starting point is when the oral taper reaches 15 mg of prednisone or its equivalent.

Changing from Oral to Inhaled Steroids

The transition from oral to inhaled corticosteroid must be closely supervised. Patients who have been maintained on oral corticosteroids for long periods or who have received frequent courses may have adrenal insufficiency. This would be less likely in patients who had been maintained on alternate-day steroids. Laboratory testing can be performed by the physician to determine the state of the adrenal gland. As the oral dosage of corticosteroid is reduced and eliminated and the inhaled steroids are utilized, it is best to assume that adrenal insufficiency exists for a period of six to twelve months after the last oral dosage has been given. If a medical illness develops, such as influenza, it is advisable to administer a dosage of oral corticosteroid that would equal what the adrenal gland would normally produce.

Intramuscular Injection of Steroids

Another method of administration of corticosteroid is by intramuscular injection. Triamcinolone acetonide is one example of a steroid that can be given on a monthly basis by this route. A recent study demonstrated that this medication could provide maintenance control equal to that achieved by oral corticosteroid. This approach may have some value in patients who find it difficult to follow a tapering oral schedule but certainly carries a high risk of total body side effects. One additional adverse effect that has been noted with intramuscular corticosteroid is atrophy or wasting of the muscle at the site of injection.

What Time Should I Take My Oral Steroid Dosage?

Because the greatest quantity of the body's corticosteroid is produced in the early morning hours it has been common practice to prescribe dosing in the morning. Patients with nocturnal asthma have often "split" the total daily dose and taken half in the morning and half at bedtime. Recent research has demonstrated that better control of asthma results from patients receiving their entire daily dosage at three P.M. This may be due partly to the slow onset of action of several hours after a dosage is ingested. This slow onset is also important when initiating treatment for a severe attack. If there is delay in the decision to give steroid this is further compounded by delayed onset of action. With the help of peak flow measurements the decision to treat should be straightforward.

Alternate-Day Steroids

Another approach to the administration of oral corticosteroid is alternate-day dosing. This approach has been found to reduce adverse effects, particularly adrenal insufficiency. Unfortunately this "day on, day off" approach is not strong enough to control the acute asthmatic attack. It may be extremely helpful, however, in maintenance control of bronchial asthma. Patients with severe disease may still experience difficulty on the "day off" and require small daily dosing for better control.

Adverse Effects of Systemic Steroids

Any adverse effects of corticosteroids are directly related to how long they are administered and in what dosage. The greater the dosage the likelier the development of side effects, especially if sustained at high dosage for a prolonged period (months to years). One of the most serious side effects is development of adrenal insufficiency. In this setting the careful administration of steroid is essential since without the patient's daily dosage there is a risk of low blood pressure and collapse. This is particularly important when the body is placed under stress as in an infection since the adrenal gland is responsible for maintaining normal body chemistry under severe conditions.

Other adverse effects of systemic corticosteroids include high blood pressure, diabetes, stomach ulcer, osteoporosis, mental changes, fluid retention, thinning of the skin with easy bruising, accelerated cataract formation, obesity, and mental changes. There may also be hormonal changes that effect the menstrual cycle. Over prolonged periods increased fat may be deposited in the liver with enlargement of this organ. All these effects are particularly damaging to the older population of asthmatics who may already have some of these problems. In these patients the underlying illness is often worsened as in the patient whose diabetes was previously controlled by diet but who on corticosteroid must now take oral medication or insulin. It is clear that in individual patients the adverse effects of oral corticosteroids may be severe and in some cases cause ailments that the patient feels are "worse than my asthma."

How Can I Avoid Side Effects of Corticosteroids?

Anytime corticosteroids are prescribed orally or by injection it must be clear that they are absolutely necessary. This is best determined by the physician in communication with the patient with readings of spirometry or peak flow. Patients should have clear guidelines from their physician concerning their use of steroids and always consult before their use. In emergencies where communication is delayed the patient should follow dosage guidelines already agreed on and report to the physician as soon as possible.

When steroids are prescribed they must be given in sufficient dosage to alleviate the attack in conjunction with other medications. One common error is to prolong treatment unnecessarily. Reducing dosage when it is appropriate reduces the magnitude of any side effects. The home monitoring by peak flow can be invaluable in deciding how often and how much of a reduction in corticosteroid is possible. If prolonged steroid use is necessary, the lowest possible but still effective dosage should be given. An alternate-day approach may also be tried.

Preparing for Side Effects

When corticosteroids are prescribed it is best to prepare for side effects, including careful monitoring of calorie intake, salt and fluid consumed in an attempt to reduce weight gain, and swelling (edema). Increased exercise, hopefully permitted by reduced asthmatic symptoms, can be extremely helpful in slowing weight gains. Exercise is important since steroids may cause myopathy or muscle weakness. Since steroids cause an increased loss of potassium from the body a diet rich in potassium is helpful. Citrus fruits and their juices as well as bananas are helpful in increasing potassium intake. Increased calcium intake with vitamin D may be helpful in reducing bone loss. In women with osteoporosis, the use of estrogen (if not contraindicated) in conjunction with calcium and vitamin D should be more effective than supplements of calcium and vitamin D alone. Patients with mild diabetes or a tendency to high blood sugar should increase restriction of their diets when they are placed on steroids. These patients must have their blood sugars closely monitored and may require treatment such as oral hypoglycemic agents or insulin.

Protecting the Stomach

Steroids should always be taken with food to minimize stomach irritation. Antacids may also be given if acidity increases but are best not taken simultaneously with the steroid since its absorption is decreased. Patients with histories of stomach ulcer are best placed on a regimen of anti-ulcer medication while they are receiving corticosteroids. This may include one of a group of medications known as H-2 antagonists that reduce the amount of stomach acid.

When Side Effects Cannot Be Prevented

Unfortunately, some effects cannot be avoided or minimized. Patients on prolonged corticosteroids should have frequent eye exams to check for accelerated formation of cataracts or increased glaucoma. There is little that can be done for the increased fragility of the skin or increased bruising other than finding the lowest maintenance dose possible or hopefully discontinuing the oral steroid successfully. The mental changes also cannot be avoided other than by lowering dosages. The initial high dosages may result in euphoria and, rarely, psychosis. Steroid withdrawal may produce depression. It is helpful to be aware of these possible effects allowing the patient and family to adjust accordingly.

Cromolyn Sodium

Cromolyn sodium, a derivative of khellin, an Egyptian herbal remedy, is a useful anti-inflammatory agent that may be used as an alternative to inhaled corticosteroids. In severe patients, cromolyn sodium (Intal) may be used in conjunction with steroids. Like the inhaled corticosteroids, cromolyn is also underused. This underutilization does not result from fear of adverse effects but rather from a misunderstanding of its application. Since its introduction cromolyn has been the drug of choice for childhood asthmatics. From this early application it has been incorrectly assumed that it was a poor drug for adults, particularly those without allergic characteristics. Many studies, however, have documented that cromolyn may be an effective drug for asthmatics of all ages, even in patients with "intrinsic" asthma. It is also clear that cromolyn does not work for all patients. Like the inhaled corticosteroids it is also slow acting and therefore requires a trial of three to six weeks to assess response. Because of this many patients abandon this drug before it has had an adequate trial.

How Does Cromolyn Work?

It is not clear how cromolyn sodium reduces inflammation. Some evidence has pointed to an action on inflammatory and allergy cells that prevents release of irritating chemicals that cause inflammation. There may also be an antagonistic action on nervous stimulation that prevents bronchoconstriction and reflex cough. Cromolyn has been demonstrated to prevent both the immediate and late reactions of asthma as well as exercise-induced asthma in many patients.

How Cromolyn Is Supplied and Used

Cromolyn sodium was initially made available as a powder for inhalation. Unfortunately, this produced considerable coughing and wheezing. It is currently also available as an aerosol for metered-dose inhaler and in solution for nebulization. When used for nebulization it may be combined with a B_2-adrenergic agonist. The recommended dosage is two puffs four times a day from a MDI or 20 mg in solution via a nebulizer, also four times a day.

Cromolyn is not an effective drug for acute asthmatic attacks and like the inhaled corticosteroids must be used as a preventive maintenance drug. For this reason cromolyn is best not started during an acute attack. It can be introduced toward the end of an oral steroid taper similar to the way that the inhaled corticosteroids are started. Also, like the inhaled corticosteroids, cromolyn can be used alone and does not necessarily require premedication with a B-adrenergic agonist.

Adverse Effects of Cromolyn

Besides being an effective drug, cromolyn has an extremely low incidence of side effects, which explains its first-line use in children where high-dose inhaled corticosteroids have been shown to slow bone development. In adults the inhaled corticosteroids are considered more effective making cromolyn a second-line agent. In those patients with adverse steroid effects cromolyn is an excellent alternative anti-inflammatory. There are few adverse effects to speak of. Occasionally, cough and wheezing may result from its inhalation. This can often be prevented with the use of a B-adrenergic agonist sprayed five to ten minutes before use or given in solution with cromolyn via nebulization. Rarely have total body effects been noted. An extremely small number of patients have noted joint pains and rash. These effects have resolved completely on discontinuation.

Nedocromil Sodium

Nedocromil sodium (Tilade) resembles cromolyn sodium in its effects as an anti-inflammatory. Nedocromil, however, is structurally different from cromolyn sodium and may also prevent the release of irritating chemicals that perpetuate the asthmatic reaction, but its mechanism of action is unknown. It also has effects on the immediate allergic response and the late phase reaction. There is some evidence that nedocromil may be helpful in reducing the number of puffs of the inhaled steroids needed to maintain good control of asthma.

How Nedocromil Is Supplied and Used

Nedocromil has been made available in the United States as an aerosol delivered by metered-dose inhaler. Compared with cromolyn sodium, nedocromil appears to be more potent and in large series of patients has been shown to be slightly more effective. The daily dosage is two puffs four times a day but may be reduced to twice a day in stable patients. Nedrocromil should be regarded as an alternative to inhaled corticosteroids and cromolyn as a preventive anti-inflammatory. It has no place in the treatment of the acute asthmatic attack and is best introduced toward the end of an oral steroid taper for patients who have suffered an acute episode. Nedocromil also has a slow onset of action and should be given for three to six weeks before judgment is made as to its effectiveness.

Adverse Effects of Nedocromil

Like cromolyn sodium, nedocromil has little total body side effects. Patient acceptance, however, has been affected by a greater incidence of nausea after its use as well as aftertaste and occasionally throat irritation. Rarely, a flushing sensation may be noted after its use. For these reasons it is unlikely that nedocromil will replace cromolyn. A menthol-flavored version is available in Europe and hopefully will be made available in the United States. It is too early to know if this will overcome some of the adverse effects noted above.

Methotrexate

Several trials of methotrexate in patients with severe, often steroid-depen-dent asthma have taken place. Methotrexate reduces the immune response of the body by reducing the number of white blood cells in tis-sues. These cells carry the irritating chemicals that can cause inflamma-tion. The use of this drug in asthma stems from its effectiveness in another inflammatory illness, rheumatoid arthritis. Patients with this severe joint disease have often benefited from low-dose (once a week) administration of methotrexate.

Early studies of methotrexate suggested this drug may have a benefi-cial effect in bronchial asthma, allowing some patients to reduce their steroid requirement. Further studies have not been as positive and long-term studies of adverse effects in asthmatic patients have not been com-pleted. Since methotrexate may cause pneumonia and scarring of the lungs known as pulmonary fibrosis, its use in patients with underlying lung disease such as asthma may prove hazardous. An additional worri-some side effect is the potential for liver damage. Patients receiving methotrexate must have frequent blood tests for liver function, chest x-rays, and comprehensive pulmonary function tests looking for evidence of fibrosis. Unless further studies show a greater benefit to this drug's use in bronchial asthma it is likely to be used sparingly.

Cyclosporin A

Other agents that suppress the immune response have also been tried in severe asthma. One of these is cyclosporin A which has been used to a great extent in preventing rejection of transplanted organs. This agent is active against lymphocytes, white blood cells that are active in asthma. Like methotrexate, studies to date do not show a great beneficial effect of cyclosporin A on asthma that would outweigh the risk of side effects on the immune system.

Other Anti-Inflammatory Agents

Gold Salts

Gold salts have been administered to asthmatic patients based on the benefit of this drug in patients with rheumatoid arthritis. Small numbers of patients have been treated with gold injections or an oral gold compound called auranofin and individual patients have been reported to reduce their symptoms and steroid requirement. Studies of large numbers of patients are lacking and this approach is not without adverse effects since gold may also cause pulmonary fibrosis. For these reasons, the use of gold salts in the treatment of asthma must be regarded as investigational.

Troleandomycin

Troleandomycin (TAO), an antibiotic, has been administered to asthmatic patients who have been steroid dependent. It appears to simply slow the excretion of one of the oral corticosteroids, methylprednisolone. Selected patients receiving methylprednisolone who are given troleandomycin have been able to reduce their steroid dosage. A similar effect of TAO has been noted on theophylline breakdown. For this reason, blood levels of theophylline are required of patients maintained on this medication during TAO administration. TAO has no anti-inflammatory effect of its own and may cause liver damage. It must be concluded that TAO has little place in the routine treatment of bronchial asthma.

Antihistamines

Antihistamines have long been regarded as contraindicated in asthmatics. This prohibition has stemmed from the drying effect antihistamines have on lung secretions and the greater potential for "plugging" of the bronchial tubes in asthmatic attacks. This adverse effect has clearly been documented in many patients. On the other hand, studies of large dosages of antihistamines in asthmatic patients have occasionally demonstrated a beneficial effect. This is not surprising since histamine is one of the irritating substances involved in provoking an asthmatic attack.

Azelastine

Azelastine is an antihistamine that has undergone trials in Japan and other countries in patients with bronchial asthma. Despite early positive results no significant benefit has been proven in large numbers of patients. One adverse effect is drowsiness. This drug is not available in the United States.

Ketotifen

Another antihistamine, Ketotifen, has been available for use in Europe for bronchial asthma. To date studies do not demonstrate a significant beneficial effect. This agent may also cause drowsiness. Until further studies of additional agents are made available there can be no basis for the routine use of antihistamines for treatment of bronchial asthma. Antihistamines may be carefully administered for nasal or sinus disease if the patient is closely monitored by a physician.

Gammaglobulin

Gammaglobulin is a protein substance that normally circulates in the blood to combat infection. A small number of severe asthmatic patients have been treated with intravenous infusions of gammaglobulin. Selected patients who received gammaglobulin have been reported to be able to reduce their steroid requirement. This treatment should be considered investigational since only a small number of patients have undergone this form of therapy.

It should be noted that gammaglobulin is often administered to patients who are born with a deficiency of this important substance. Often these patients experience frequent infections that may affect the sinuses and bronchial tubes. Some of these patients also have bronchial asthma and treatment of the gammaglobulin deficiency may actually result in improvement of the asthmatic condition. This "replacement therapy" differs from the investigational use of gammaglobulin in bronchial asthma noted above.

Are Asthma Medications Addictive?

Many patients fear they will become addicted to their asthma medications and be unable to stop their use. This may partly be due to dependence on medication for the relief of symptoms and attacks. This fear of addiction may explain why some patients do not take their medications.

There is no evidence of the development of addiction to asthma medications. When good control of asthma is achieved it is often possible to reduce or discontinue medication that is no longer needed. However, good control must come first since withdrawal of medication may result in increased frequency of attacks.

Adrenal Insufficiency

In the case of systemic corticosteroids, the management of reduction and withdrawal of these agents must be closely supervised in view of possible adrenal insufficiency. Patients with severe asthma may become "steroid dependent" for control of their disease but that does not represent an addiction to medication.

Are There Delayed Effects of Asthma Medications?

Another concern of patients is whether long-term use of asthma drugs will have serious adverse effects, another reason why patients may reduce or eliminate medications on their own.

Long-term use in adults of the B-agonists, theophylline, cromolyn sodium, and inhaled corticosteroids have not shown any evidence of delayed adverse effects. In children, inhaled corticosteroids may have adverse effects on growth and bone development. These agents may still be necessary, however, when the risk of severe, uncontrolled asthma outweighs the possible detrimental effects on bone growth. Nedocromil and ipra-tropium bromide are still relatively new and long-term experience with these agents is forthcoming. At this time there is no evidence of possible delayed adverse effects of these agents.

Oral Corticosteroids

In both children and adults, long-term effects of the oral corticosteroids must be anticipated. These effects are outlined above and must be weighed against the dangers of uncontrolled asthma. Once systemic steroids are required there should be frequent review of their necessity with the goal of reducing dosage or withdrawal if possible. Alternate-day administration should always be considered if patients must remain on oral corticosteroids.

How Should Asthma Drugs Be Used?

In this chapter specific asthma medications have been discussed. As their number and effectiveness increases, confusion has also increased as to how these medications should be taken. Patients are often given several different medications and may find it difficult to use them all. Many patients complain they are "overmedicated" and stop medications on their own. Chapter 5 provides a strategy for using asthma medications effectively.

CHAPTER 5

Strategy for Medication Treatment

TREATING asthma requires a step-by-step approach in order to provide the correct medication. This "step therapy" also ensures that medication will be given in the proper dosage and that unnecessary medication will not be given. To prescribe the correct asthma medication, a physician must grade patients according to the severity of their condition. This chapter will define asthma in terms of its severity and proposes a strategy for treatment based on degree of severity.

Adult Asthma: Mild, Moderate, and Severe

Mild asthma is defined as a condition in which attacks do not occur more than twice a week and never during sleep. Between attacks, peak flow rates are maintained at the patient's "personal best." Moderate to severe asthmatics experience more than two attacks a week, use their bronchodilators daily and often have nocturnal symptoms. Severe asthmatics require regular bronchodilator use, often need oral corticosteroid courses, have been hospitalized for severe attacks usually with assisted respiration, and they often have night attacks. Steroid-dependent asthmatics form a subgroup of these severe patients. These patients are never without oral corticosteroids due to almost continuous symptoms.

Use Severity Definitions Cautiously

These severity definitions are helpful but should not be employed rigidly. Patients with allergic or extrinsic asthma may only be symptomatic during certain seasons depending on the amount of pollen to which they are exposed. Some allergic patients experience symptoms only when exposed to certain allergens like cat dander; others may display symptoms only during an upper respiratory tract infection like a sore throat or sinus infection. A few patients will be symptomatic only after exercise. All these patients could also be defined as mild asthmatics even though their attacks may sometimes be severe. To be sure, asthma severity varies from patient to patient and strict definitions are not easily applied.

Strategy for Treatment: Step Therapy

All patients should have a strategy for treatment that they have discussed and agreed to after consulting with their physician. It is best that these instructions be in writing for easy reference and that close communication (aided by peak flow measurements) be maintained with the physician. Often the details of a "strategy" will be revised. No treatment plan should ever be regarded as final since there are frequent variations in asthma as well as new medications that become available. Treatment is best given in a "step-by-step" fashion, avoiding simultaneous administration of several new agents, so the physician and patient can more accurately determine what treatment is most effective.

Treatment Goals

Treatment goals for bronchial asthma are maintaining a normal lifestyle including vigorous exercise, reversing bronchial narrowing, inflammation and irritability thereby sustaining "normal" lung function and avoiding adverse medication effects. Symptoms such as shortness of breath, wheezing, and coughing should be minimal. Whenever medication side effects like those encountered with long-term oral corticosteroids outweigh benefits the medication program must be revised.

Treatment Strategy: Mild Asthma

As a rule a mild asthmatic can often be treated with infrequent use of a B_2-adrenergic agonist delivered by MDI. The B-agonist would be used "as needed," not regularly. Short-acting agents are preferred because of their more rapid onset. Inflammation in the bronchial tubes is sometimes present in this group of patients. Because there are infrequent symptoms and little pulmonary function test abnormality a strong case for an anti-inflammatory agent cannot be made. Remember, anti-inflammatory agents usually require regular and prolonged use. Some patients with allergic seasonal asthma, however, may start an anti-inflammatory agent (inhaled corticosteroid, cromolyn, or nedocromil) two to three weeks before the start of their "allergy season" and continue it for two to three consecutive months while maintaining their B-agonist as needed. For example, patients in the northeastern United States who are sensitive to tree and grass pollen may want to start an anti-inflammatory agent on April 1st while those with ragweed allergy should begin on August 1st.

There is some controversy regarding treatment of patients with mild bronchial asthma. Some physicians advocate regular, daily use of an anti-inflammatory agent in addition to "as needed" B_2-agonist. A recent study of patients receiving a corticosteroid (budesonide) spray demonstrated that when the medication was withdrawn asthma symptoms increased and lung function tests deteriorated. Although this study demonstrates the effectiveness of inhaled corticosteroids in treatment of bronchial asthma, it does not establish the need for this therapy in patients with mild asthma.

Treatment Strategy: Moderate Asthma

Patients with moderate asthma should continue to use a B_2-adrenergic agonist aerosol but must add an anti-inflammatory agent. This combination would be considered first-line therapy. The anti-inflammatory agent of choice for adults is a topically active inhaled corticosteroid. Cromolyn and nedocromil would be good alternatives and may occasionally be considered first-line drugs in cough asthma where blockage of bronchial nerve reflexes often helps to reduce symptoms. Cromolyn is also preferred in children and during pregnancy. By adding an anti-inflammatory agent, patients in this group are often less symptomatic and can usually reduce overuse of B-agonist.

In moderate asthma, a long-acting B-agonist may be particularly helpful. This agent is administered every twelve hours on a regular basis. Patients who receive a long-acting B-agonist spray may still need a short-acting agent when symptoms break through. This has been appropriately termed "rescue" medication. Adding a long-acting B-agonist, however, frequently results in a reduction in the use of the short-acting agent. In view of the detrimental effects of overuse of B-agonists, this reduction is highly beneficial. Due to the slow onset of action, it must be emphasized that the long-acting B-agonist must not be used for relief of acute asthmatic attacks.

The Next Step in Moderate Asthma

Patients in the moderate group who are still symptomatic with reduced activity and flow rates despite the combination of B_2-adrenergic agonist and an anti-inflammatory agent will require additional second-line therapy. For bronchodilatation, adding an oral preparation of the B-agonist, theophylline and/or ipratropium bromide may be helpful. Those with nocturnal symptoms may respond to evening administration of a long-acting B-agonist or theophylline. If attacks continue to be frequent a trial of an additional anti-inflammatory agent would be the next step. If the patient has been receiving an inhaled corticosteroid then cromolyn or nedocromil may be added. It should be emphasized again that the decision to start or stop medications should be based on objective findings (spirometry or peak flow readings) in addition to the patient's symptoms and frequency of attacks.

Treatment Strategy: Moderate to Severe Asthma

Patients with moderate to severe asthma often need courses of oral corticosteroids when they continue to experience attacks and have lowered flow rates despite maximal first- and second-line therapy. It is always helpful before starting oral corticosteroids to review the correct use of MDI sprays as well as to emphasize the use and benefit of a spacer. Discussions between patient and physician must be frequent in this group to reiterate individual goals of treatment and to discuss the potential side effects of oral corticosteroids. Often it will become clear that a medication (usually inhaled corticosteroid) has not been used due to fear of dependency or side effects. When these questions are answered satisfactorily, resumption of this medication may avoid the use of oral steroids and their side effects.

TABLE 4. STEP-BY-STEP STRATEGY FOR TREATMENT OF ASTHMA

Mild Asthma

Inhaled B_2-Agonist As Needed

Moderate Asthma

Add an Inhaled Anti-Inflammatory Agent:
Corticosteroid / Cromolyn / Nedocromil

Use Long-Acting Inhaled B_2-Agonist Every 12 Hours
(Use Short-Acting B_2-Agonist for 'Rescue' from Acute Attack)

Severe Asthma

Use High-Dose Inhaled Corticosteroid

Long-Acting Inhaled B2-Agonist Every 12 Hours
(Short-Acting B_2-Agonist for 'Rescue')

Add Theophylline or Inhaled Anticholinergic

The Next Step: Oral Corticosteroids

Treatment Strategy: Severe Asthma

In the patient with severe asthma a home nebulizer should be considered. This device may be used to deliver not only a B_2-adrenergic agonist but also cromolyn sodium. This combined aerosol therapy may be extremely helpful in certain patients. A nebulizer may not prove more advantageous than medication delivered by MDI for every patient.

Severe Asthma: the Next Step

In the severe asthmatic who is maintained on maximal first- and second-line therapy and requires frequent courses of corticosteroid, maintenance oral steroid may also be necessary. This should always be given in the smallest dose that is effective and only after a trial of alternate-day therapy. Those patients who need more than 10 mg of prednisone (or its equivalent) for maintenance with significant side effects like osteoporosis should be considered candidates for trials of steroid-sparing anti-inflammatory agents like methotrexate. Discussion of potential reactions and success rates of these agents must take place before initiating this third-line therapy.

The Peak Flow Meter and the Acute Attack

As outlined in chapter 3, peak flow meter readings may be used to direct the management of an acute asthmatic attack. The patient's strategy for treatment should include peak flow meter readings. The patient and physician should design a plan of treatment based largely on peak flow measurements. Once the patient has obtained a "personal best" value, changes in this "normal" reading can be used to direct therapy. Changes in peak flow of 25 percent, 50 percent, and 75 percent are useful guidelines for assessing the severity of an attack and how the patient should respond. To avoid serious episodes, treatment should be initiated at the earliest indication of an attack (25 percent decrease in peak flow).

Oral corticosteroids should be used for significant drops in flow (50 percent decrease). Emergency medical attention should be given for severe decreases (75 percent drop in peak flow). Table 5 is an example of a plan of action for acute asthmatic attacks.

Childhood Asthma

In evaluating the childhood asthmatic the physician must rely more on the patient's history and physical findings since measurements of pulmonary function may be difficult to obtain. This is particularly true for children under five years of age. Children older than five are generally able to provide peak flow measurements.

**TABLE 5.   PLAN OF TREATMENT FOR ACUTE ATTACKS
BASED ON PEAK FLOW MEASUREMENTS**

Measure Peak Flow Twice a Day
Obtain 'Personal Best' Value

If Peak Flow Falls by 25 Percent
Use B_2-Agonist for Immediate Relief
If Improvement Not Maintained Increase Inhaled Steroid

If Peak Flow Falls by 50 Percent
Use B_2-Agonist for Immediate Relief
Begin Course of Oral Corticosteroid
Inform Physician

If Peak Flow Falls by 75 Percent
Use B_2-Agonist for Immediate Relief
Begin Oral Corticosteroid and Seek Medical Attention

The Medical History

In the child's history the physician should look for evidence of cough and wheezing. Changes in a child's activity may reflect shortness of breath especially if there is difficulty during exercise. Awakening at night may reflect nocturnal asthma. As in adults the presence of nasal symptoms (drip, sneezing, congestion) may signal an allergy and increase the likelihood of asthma. A strong family history of allergy or asthma may help identify the childhood asthmatic.

The Physical Examination

The physical examination of an asthmatic child does not greatly differ from that performed on the adult. Once again the presence of wheezing does not confirm the diagnosis. In a child there is a greater incidence of foreign body aspiration which may produce wheezing and mimic asthma. Cystic fibrosis must be considered in a child with cough, sputum production, and wheezing. As in the adult patient wheezing may be absent or intermittent.

Asthma in Infants

Asthma may occur in infants. More than half of childhood patients developed their first symptoms before age two. The most common source of asthma in children six months of age or younger is viral infection. This is often viral bronchitis or pneumonia. Indications of asthma in this age group may be a change in the child's cry or ability to feed or suckle. Children breathe rapidly but an increase in this rate or change in skin color due to a lack of oxygen called cyanosis may be significant indicators of asthma. Since the physician is unable to rely on measurements of airflow to determine the severity of asthma in this young age group measurement of blood oxygen is often necessary.

Treatment Strategy: Mild Childhood Asthma

In mild childhood asthma the initial treatment is use of the B_2-adrenergic agonist. Due to difficulty using MDIs in younger patients (under age five)

there must be increased reliance on nebulized medication and oral preparations (tablets or elixirs). A trial of the powder form of a B-agonist such as
albuterol may be easier for a child to use than a metered-dose inhaler. Use
of a MDI with a spacer with facemask attachment may be particularly
helpful in young patients to ensure better delivery of aerosol medication.
As with adult patients there is a greater chance of side effects (nervousness, tremor) in a child receiving oral or nebulized medication.

Treatment Strategy: Moderate Childhood Asthma

Children with moderate asthma experiencing more than two attacks a
week should have additional therapy added to the B-agonist. Cromolyn
provides an excellent choice for an anti-inflammatory agent in the childhood asthmatic due to absence of total body effects. It is approved for children age five and older with insufficient data for younger patients.
Cromolyn is available for nebulizer use, which may be more suitable for
younger patients as well as a MDI. Nedocromil has been approved for children age twelve and older and is only currently available as a MDI. It
should soon be approved for children six to twelve years of age as well. In
a child these agents should be considered first-line choices.

Moderate to Severe Childhood Asthma: the Next Step

Inhaled Corticosteroid

Childhood asthmatics not well controlled on cromolyn or nedocromil
(moderate to severe asthma) should receive additional anti-inflammatory
therapy as an inhaled corticosteroid. These agents, however, have been
found to affect bone growth and adrenal metabolism in children in
dosages above 400 ug per day but are considered safe up to this dosage.
The side effects of using higher dosages of inhaled corticosteroids in children should be weighed against the effects of uncontrolled asthma. There
is insufficient data on the use of the inhaled corticosteroids in children
below the age of six.

Theophylline

Theophylline should be considered for use in the childhood asthmatic who is uncontrolled on the primary therapy of the B-agonist and cromolyn or nedocromil. Unfortunate side effects such as nervousness, however, limit its usefulness. Recent studies have raised the question of a learning disability that may be attributed to theophylline. Additional adverse effects are stomach upset and headache. As in adults, blood levels must be monitored to ensure an effective therapeutic level.

Anticholingergic Agents

The anticholinergic agent, ipratropium bromide, may be used in children age twelve and older as a second- or third-line agent. Since most childhood asthmatics are allergic it is not likely that this agent would provide significant bronchodilatation. It is available in a nebulizer form as well as a MDI.

Treatment Strategy: Severe Childhood Asthma

Severe childhood asthmatics may require oral corticosteroids if they are not controlled with first- and second-line therapy. These patients continue to have several attacks a week and reduced airflows despite maximal therapy. The adverse effects are similar to those of adults but are more significant in regard to growth and bone development in the youngest patients. Alternate-day therapy should be attempted for patients who require maintenance therapy due to severe disease.

The National Asthma Education Program Report

The National Heart, Lung and Blood Institute (NHLB) and its National Asthma Education Program (NAEP) convened a panel of experts on the management of asthma who released a comprehensive report ("Guidelines for the Diagnosis and Management of Asthma") in 1991. This excellent resource included a suggestion for a "traffic light system" that would allow patients to easily remember how to manage their asthma. This green-yellow-red zone system has been adopted by many physicians and has been included in at least one peak flow meter design.

The Green Zone

As defined by the NAEP the green zone is a safe area in which the asthma patient experiences few or no symptoms. Peak flow measurements are 80–100 percent of a patient's predicted normal value or personal best with no more than a 20 percent swing in values. Medications are individualized for each patient, whether they are mild, moderate, or severe asthmatics.

The Yellow Zone

The yellow zone outlined by the NAEP "signals caution." The patient has peak flows that are 50–80 percent of their predicted normal or personal best and/or asthma symptoms that may include nocturnal attacks, coughing, wheezing, decreased activity, and chest tightness. This "zone" indicates that medications should be adjusted according to the management plan suggested by the physician. Patients who make frequent visits to the yellow zone should have their maintenance medications reviewed and adjusted.

The Red Zone

The red zone signals a "medical alert." Peak flows are below 50 percent of the predicted value or personal best and asthma symptoms are frequent, including at rest. The patient's management plan should immediately be put into place for this degree of attack as previously outlined. Typically, this calls for immediate use of a B-agonist and introduction of oral corticosteroids. Patients who do not respond require immediate medical attention, usually an emergency room visit. Patients who fall into the red zone should certainly have their maintenance asthma program reviewed and adjusted.

Should this Terminology Be Used?

The simple terminology suggested by the NAEP may be helpful to patients in managing their asthma. For anyone familiar with traffic signals, it is certainly easy to remember. Peak flow meters with green-yellow-red colored scales or stickers are available. Remember, however, that treatment decisions should be based on prior consultation with the physician and the patient's record of personal best flows and not by color zones alone. Each patient should have green, yellow, and red zones defined with written guidelines for treatment decisions.

Putting Your Strategy to Work

In this chapter asthma has been defined as mild, moderate, and severe and specific treatment strategies proposed for each category. A system based on traffic signal colors has been introduced. Whatever strategy is used for the treatment of asthma, its success depends on a working partnership between patient and physician. Up to this point the physician has directed treatment and provided guidelines. The next chapter discusses the patient's role in treatment.

CHAPTER 6

How to Participate in Managing Your Asthma

FOR an asthma treatment strategy to succeed, the patient must be an active participant. Patients who take an active role in their care have better control over their disease. The health benefit from patient participation can be applied to any illness but seems particularly true in diseases like asthma and diabetes. Patients who participate in their own care are better educated in regard to their illness and communicate well with their physicians. These characteristics are extremely important in managing bronchial asthma. This chapter discusses the steps patients can take to become active participants in their care and specific suggestions are offered regarding diet, stress, and work.

Self-Monitoring and Education

In managing bronchial asthma a patient can play an active role in decision making by closely monitoring airflows with a home peak flow meter. The peak flow meter is described in chapter 3. From the record of the peak flows a physician can judge the effectiveness of treatment, evaluate the patient's response to new drugs, pinpoint adverse environmental influences at home and work, and determine the need for emergency management. Peak flows may also be used for special situations such as before and after exercise to determine a patient's response to various asthma triggers.

Your physician should be your primary source of information. Limits on time may prevent discussion of all-important issues on an initial visit, so make a list of important topics you want to discuss so you can raise these issues during follow-up visits. Ask your doctor about recommended reading to further your education. Before leaving the physician's office you should have been taught the correct use of a MDI, peak flow meter, and spacer if they are prescribed. Ask lots of questions. Videotapes of proper inhalation techniques for using MDIs are available. Written instructions on the use of your medications should be given to you. "What are the side effects I should be aware of?" "Are there any drug interactions with my other medicines?" are excellent questions you should ask.

At home keep a record of your doctor office visits and appointments. A diary of your peak flow measurements should also be maintained. Mark your calendar when you started using a MDI so you can mark ahead the date when it should be refilled. Always carry a list of your medications with you as well as a fresh bronchodilator spray for emergency use. If you travel, carry a set of your prescriptions in case your medication is mislaid. Research the climate you will be traveling to as well as important aspects of the locale such as local allergens or the altitude. Ask your physician about the effects of altitude on your condition and whether you should have prescriptions for emergency medications such as antibiotics or corticosteroids.

Choosing Your Asthma Physician

Many types of physicians administer treatment to patients with bronchial asthma. Family physicians, internists, allergists, and pulmonologists are all involved in treatment of patients with asthma. Excellent care may be provided by any of these types of physicians who are well trained and experienced in treatment of asthma. An asthma specialist is often a physician who has specialty training in asthma as well as other chest diseases, such as a pulmonologist. Patients with unstable asthma or disease that is unresponsive to treatment should certainly be seen by an asthma specialist who can work in concert with the primary physician. Even patients with mild disease may benefit from a specialist's review of their diagnosis and treatment. Patients with asthma should undergo an allergy evaluation, which may be administered under the direction of an allergist.

Many factors enter into your choice of a physician in addition to training and expertise. It should be apparent to each patient if the "chemistry is right" and that a good rapport has been established with a physician. How the physician responds to questions and listens to concerns about chronic disease, fears of medication effects, and descriptions of side effects should make it clear if the right choice of a physician has been made. Other important considerations are availability, how emergency calls are handled, as well as access to facilities for evaluation and treatment. Finally, the patient must feel that a partnership has been established with the physician for achieving the best possible care.

Reducing Allergens at Home and Work

The patient can take an active role in managing the environment at home and in the office. In allergic patients avoiding offending allergen(s) may drastically reduce the frequency of asthmatic attacks. Allergens can be identified through a history of reaction and skin or blood testing. Common allergens are dust mites, mold spores, animal dander, and plant pollens. Insects such as the cockroach may also produce allergens that precipitate attacks. Specific allergens may be identified through testing of samples taken from the home. See appendix A for more information on collecting samples.

Dust Mites

Dust mites may play a significant role in many asthmatic attacks. These extremely small insects depend on moisture for survival and live on human skin dander. They have been found in abundant quantities in mattresses, pillows, clothes, bed coverings, carpets, towels, and even stuffed animals. In the home the highest concentrations have been found in the bedroom. It is the feces of the dust mite that produces an allergic reaction.

Because these droppings are airborne when dust is disturbed they can be inhaled and cause allergic reactions. The particles are large enough to be trapped, however, and the patient can significantly reduce the number of dust mites through specific measures.

These measures include trapping dust mites by using a zippered mattress and pillow cover. Sheets and bed covers should be washed weekly in hot water. Carpeting should be removed wherever possible and remaining carpeting treated with a chemical agent (acaracide) such as benzyl benzoate (Acarosan) or tannic acid that kills mites. See appendix A for more information on obtaining these materials. Vacuuming is important and should be done once a week, preferably not by the asthma patient. If you must vacuum yourself use a dust mask and a vacuum cleaner with high-density paper bags and filtration as well as a HEPA filter (High Efficiency Particulate Air). Indoor humidity levels should be reduced to less than 50 percent with a dehumidifier.

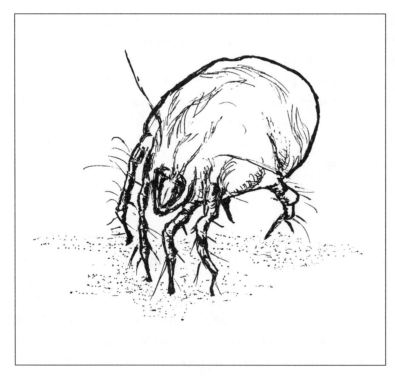

Figure 20.
The Dust Mite
(Enlarged)

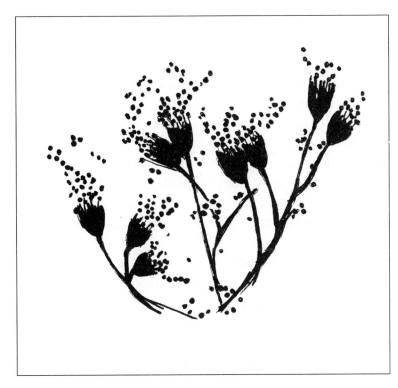

Figure 21.
Penicillium Mold

An air filter may be helpful in reducing allergen levels for the dust mite as well as other offending substances. Air filters may be mechanical or electrical. One of the best mechanical types incorporates a HEPA filter. These come in various sizes according to the volume of the room (amount of air) that has to be filtered and circulated. Know the dimensions of the room in which the air filter will be placed before you purchase one. One example of an electrical filter is the electrostatic precipitator. These filters and the HEPA filter can be placed in a central forced air system in the home. Electrical filters require more frequent cleaning than mechanical types.

Molds

Molds are fungi that grow well in warm and moist environments. They are frequently found in the bathroom, kitchen, and basement of homes. Airborne mold spores are the allergens that can produce asthmatic attacks in sensitive individuals. Many steps can be taken to reduce mold spores in the home in addition to the air filter and vacuum cleaner discussed above. This step includes reducing mold growth by lowering humidity levels to 25–50 percent with a dehumidifier. Remember that the dehumidifier must be cleaned and emptied regularly.

Mold growth is highest in warmer months, so an air conditioner can be extremely helpful. Attention must be paid to preventing contamination of the air conditioner itself since any moist area may promote mold growth. Remember the automobile air conditioner, too. Many patients describe allergy and asthma symptoms each time they use their car's air conditioner due to its exposure to mold. Ventilation is important to reduce mold spore inhalation. An exhaust fan in the bathroom and kitchen to reduce humidity levels is also helpful. Chemical sprays are available to kill mold and prevent its regrowth in areas that are highly susceptible (showers, basements, air conditioners, etc.). Appendix A contains useful information on obtaining these materials. An asthmatic patient should avoid any chemical spray that produces a strong odor, however, and this type of spraying is best done by someone else. Everyone using chemical sprays should use a facemask and make sure there is plenty of ventilation. Houseplants are not a major source of mold spores but are best kept to a minimum since they increase humidity levels. Spores may also be liberated when the plants are potted or watered.

Animal Allergens

Animal allergens are potent triggers of allergic and asthmatic attacks and are commonly found in homes with pets. These allergens may also be present in homes or offices where animals are not kept since they can stick to clothing and be carried to any location by the pet's owner. The allergens consist of dander and saliva and are not related to breed or coat length. All breeds of cats, for example, share a common allergen, which may be airborne or present in mattresses, carpets, bed covers, and pillows. As in the control of dust mites and mold spores an air filter can be extremely helpful.

The best way to reduce animal allergens is to get rid of the animal. Restricting a pet to a certain room or a portion of the home does not prevent airborne particles from spreading throughout the home. Even after the pet has been removed allergens may remain for several months. Cleaning with 3 percent tannic acid solution can denature residual animal allergen. Cat allergen has been demonstrated to remain for years at significant levels in mattresses. A mattress and pillow cover will be helpful in encasing animal allergens. If a pet must remain in the home several additional steps are also helpful. Washing a cat weekly will reduce dander levels. This will be difficult at first but cats can be gradually introduced to bathing by starting with one area at a time. The animal's coat can be treated with a spray or solution that reduces exposure to allergens (see appendix A). Do not forget small pets like birds and rodents that may produce severe asthmatic attacks in sensitive individuals.

Reducing Indoor Pollution

Asthma attacks may be precipitated indoors by airborne irritants that are not allergens. In the home commonly found irritants include tobacco smoke, strong odors, pollutants from gas stoves, wood stoves, and fireplaces.

Active Smoking

Patients with asthma who smoke do not have to look far to find a reason to stop. Cigarette smoking is the leading cause of respiratory illness and death in the United States. All of these illnesses and deaths are preventable. Cigarette smoking may cause permanent damage in the lung leading to emphysema and chronic bronchitis. It should be clear to the individual with asthma who smokes that this habit may change a reversible disease (asthma) to an irreversible and often fatal disease (emphysema). In addition, cigarette smoking has been shown to increase "irritability" of the bronchial tubes and may therefore be a considered cause of asthma. It has been documented that smoking affects the immune system and the defense of the lung against infection. Smokers have higher rates of sinus and bronchial infection than do nonsmokers. These infections may trigger asthmatic attacks.

Despite these facts and many others that link cigarette smoking to cancer of the lung and other organs, many patients with asthma continue to smoke. Some stop during attacks and resume when they feel better.

How to Stop Smoking

There is no foolproof method of stopping, but some measures have proved helpful. A patient should work closely with a physician, reviewing pulmonary function tests that may already show permanent changes, supporting the decision to quit. It also helps to review the benefits of stopping. Studies have documented that patients who stop smoking have a marked reduction in cough, wheezing, expectoration, and shortness of breath. This may occur as soon as one month after stopping. Reports also show that there are fewer infections and improvement in pulmonary function tests after smoking cessation. It is often helpful to demonstrate with a peak flow meter that smoking one cigarette can produce a drop in air movement. The next step is to set a "stop date." It can also help to sign a stop-smoking contract with the physician.

A great deal of information has documented the powerful addictive properties of nicotine. Your physician can help you assess the degree of physical addiction and the role of psychological dependence. For patients with physical addiction, replacement therapy with nicotine in the form of a chewing gum or patch may be helpful. Other measures can be recommended if this is not successful. A psychological dependence can also be treated successfully. In every patient the message must be clear: "You must stop smoking."

Environmental Tobacco Smoke

Nonsmokers are exposed to many of the same injurious agents inhaled by active smokers. The dangers of second-hand tobacco smoke have been widely publicized. Among them it should be noted that children exposed to parental second-hand smoke have been found to have more respiratory illnesses, including asthma. Asthmatic children of smokers have been shown to have more frequent attacks. The Environmental Protection Agency (EPA) has reported a higher frequency of asthmatic attacks in up to one million children of cigarette smokers. In the same report the EPA attributed up to 300,000 cases of bronchitis and other respiratory infections in small children to their exposure to second-hand smoke. Environmental tobacco smoke is one of the most frequent triggers of asthmatic attacks reported by patients. In sensitive individuals, even brief inhalation of second-hand smoke may precipitate a severe asthmatic attack.

Asthmatic individuals frequently report that household family members continue to smoke despite the patient's illness. Often the smoking

TABLE 6.   TIPS FOR ALLERGY-PROOFING YOUR HOME OR OFFICE

To Reduce Dust Mites

Remove carpets, rugs, upholstered furniture

Encase mattresses, pillows, and box springs in zippered covers

Wash sheets and bedding in hot water weekly

Wash stuffed animals

Use a HEPA air filter

To Reduce Mold

Keep humidity levels at 30–50 percent with a dehumidifier

Use a mold remover spray on bathroom and basement walls,
window sills, air conditioners, humidifiers, plant soil

Remove carpeting over concrete floors

Use a HEPA air filter

To Reduce Indoor Pollution

Ban smoking from your home; avoid gas and wood stoves, fireplaces

Avoid cooking odors with an exhaust fan; paint fumes

Use air conditioner, HEPA filter to keep out pollens, particulates, fumes individual will report that they only smoke "in another room." Separating smokers and nonsmokers in the home or workplace does not eliminate exposure to second-hand smoke. To reduce exposure smoking must be completely prohibited or restricted to a separately ventilated area in order to provide protection for all nonsmokers and especially those with bronchial asthma.

Wood Smoke

Wood smoke from wood-burning stoves and fireplaces may also be an irritant and aggravate bronchial asthma. Approximately 6 percent of homes in the United States have wood stoves and 19 percent have fireplaces. Although the smoke from wood stoves and fireplaces is vented to the outdoors, emissions are found to contaminate indoor air during start-up and when stoking. Particulate matter may also be produced from these sources which may irritate bronchial asthma. Good ventilation is essential and an air filter will be helpful if a stove cannot be removed.

Gas Stoves

Gas stoves may also be a source of indoor pollution. Several airborne irritants may be released by gas combustion including nitrogen dioxide. Although some studies have not found an association between gas stoves and asthma, a recent report suggests that gas stoves may aggravate asthma. As a rule, asthmatic patients should avoid gas and wood-burning stoves.

Formaldehyde and Other Indoor Pollutants

Formaldehyde and other compounds that exist as vapors are found indoors as emissions from construction materials, furnishings like carpeting, and insulation. Formaldehyde is used in many products including cosmetics, toiletries, medications, and in some foods as a preservative. This compound is known to be irritating to the lining of the nose and bronchial tubes and cases of occupational asthma due to formaldehyde have been reported. At this time, it is not clear how great a role formaldehyde and similar compounds play in aggravating bronchial asthma. To minimize your risk of exposure to these vapors, building materials and furnishings can be selected that do not contain formaldehyde and that have low rates of emission of similar compounds. Ventilation can be increased in areas that are suspected or known to have increased amounts of these substances. Existing sources of formaldehyde such as carpeting can be removed from the home or office. Cleaning solutions, gasoline, and similar materials are best stored in a separate area with excellent ventilation.

Asthmatic attacks have been demonstrated to occur frequently when patients are exposed to strong odors. Simple cooking odors may be extremely irritating. Household sprays, especially those used for cleaning, are often sources of irritation. Other examples include insecticide sprays, deodorants, hair sprays, and perfumes. Paint fumes can be extremely irritating and should be avoided. The simple measures of ensuring adequate ventilation and using an air filter will provide relief from many of these odors if they cannot be avoided.

Ozone and Other Air Pollutants

Air pollutants such as ozone and sulfur dioxide may be found in the home. The levels of these gases are lower indoors than outdoors but still may be irritating to patients with asthma and other lung diseases. Fine particle pollutants may also be found in the home. Patients should be aware of pollution levels and air pollution "alerts" issued by local public health authorities. Air conditioning can be effective in reducing irritating airborne gases. An air filter reduces levels of particulate pollutants.

Outdoor Allergens and Irritants

Avoidance

Avoidance is the best way to reduce your number of asthmatic attacks triggered by exposure to pollens, molds, and other outdoor allergens. Sensitive individuals are best protected in an air-conditioned environment that contains an air filter. Pollen and mold spore counts are commonly found in newspapers and TV weather reports.

Pollens and Molds

Pollens are seasonal and patients should be able to prepare ahead for particularly difficult months. Patients with known tree pollen allergy who are symptomatic in the spring, for example, may reduce the frequency of asthma attacks by beginning an anti-inflammatory agent such as inhaled corticosteroid or cromolyn or nedocromil two to three weeks before the start of their "season." Those who are sensitive to grasses and ragweed will want to maintain their medication through to the first frost.

Mold spores are more plentiful in warmer months. Thousands of different species of mold exist. They may be found in high numbers on both dry and rainy days. Alternaria is a mold often found in dry, warm climates and in farming areas. Fusarium mold is often found in plants and is abundant during damp, humid weather. Other molds are found in decaying wood and soil. Be sure you anticipate exposure during outdoor activities (mowing the lawn, raking leaves). A simple filter mask may help you reduce your exposure. Patients may also reduce exposure by staying indoors, using air conditioning and air filtration.

Air Pollution

Air pollution has been demonstrated to have significant adverse effects on patients with lung disease and especially those with bronchial asthma. The Environmental Protection Agency (EPA) has set standards for most common pollutants, including sulfur dioxide (SO_2), nitrogen dioxide (NO_2), carbon monoxide, ozone, particulates, and lead. Sulfur dioxide and particulates are produced by combustion of sulfur-containing fuels like coal and petroleum. Sulfur dioxide is found in high concentrations near steel mills, power plants, and other factories that burn coal or oil. Particulates are the soot and ashes produced by incinerators, smokestacks, and diesel trucks.

Nitrogen dioxide is a product of industry found in high concentrations when fuel is burned and it may be released by power plants and automobiles. This type of industrial pollution affects primarily the central and eastern United States but may also be found in any area with many vehicles. Carbon monoxide is also emitted by automobiles and factories.

Asthmatics are extremely sensitive to sulfur dioxide and may react to exposure with constriction of the bronchial tubes to increased levels of this gas in outdoor air. Increased levels of particulate pollution have also been associated with exacerbations of chronic respiratory disease. The effect of particulate pollution depends on the size and chemical nature of the inhaled particles. The smaller particles have a greater likelihood of reaching the lungs of patients with asthma, bronchitis, and emphysema. A recent study links particulate pollution with a greater likelihood of death from respiratory disease.

Photochemical pollution or "smog" is the product of the action of sunlight on vehicle exhaust and chemical fumes. Ozone is a product of this interaction and can be used as an index for this type of pollution. Southern California was the first area affected by photochemical pollution but it has become common in major cities throughout the United States, especially in the summer. Ozone has been shown to cause a reduction in lung function in normal subjects and individuals with asthma. It has been suggested that prolonged exposure may produce chronic lung disease.

National standards for air pollutants have been set with a "margin of safety" that should protect the health of patients with asthma and other illnesses as well as the general population. Air pollution "alerts" are issued by local public health agencies when increased levels of pollution are noted. Air pollutants will be found in greater amounts when weather conditions produce stagnant air circulation. The warm summer months in the eastern United States are particularly dangerous due to increased ozone levels. Patients are advised to stay indoors in an air-conditioned environment during periods of increased pollution. Exercise outdoors, which increases the likelihood of inhaling pollutants, should especially be avoided during these periods. Remember that pollutants like ozone may also be damaging to individuals with normal lungs and therefore should be avoided by everyone.

Air Temperature

Patients should also consider air temperature. Cold air is extremely irritating in patients with bronchial asthma and may produce severe attacks. Individuals with asthma appear to warm cold air less quickly and effi-

ciently than non-asthmatics. This warming takes place in the large air passages of the nose, sinuses, throat, and windpipe. One simple measure
patients should take is to wrap the face with a scarf that warms air before
it is inhaled. A cold air mask is commercially available (see appendix A)
and may provide more protection in the winter.

How to Avoid Severe or Fatal Asthma Attacks

Patients who experience severe or near-fatal asthma attacks must be
active participants in monitoring and managing their asthma. Several
characteristics of fatal or near-fatal asthma attacks stand out and I emphasize them.

There is usually a period of falling airflows and increased wheezing,
cough, and shortness of breath that precedes a severe attack. In this critical time the introduction of oral corticosteroid or an adjustment of maintenance treatment may prevent a near-fatal asthma attack. Unfortunately,
patients with severe and subsequently fatal asthma often experience
denial of their condition and symptoms. These patients are particularly
vulnerable to fatal attacks since they often disregard instructions to monitor flows and take medications. Usually, these patients admit to self-med-
ication without communication with the physician, lowering dosages or
omitting entirely oral and inhaled corticosteroids (for fear of side effects
despite a life-threatening disease), and by reducing the number of sprays
from the recommended dosages of B-agonists, cromolyn, and nedocromil.

It is not clear why these patients place themselves at greater risk
through denial of their disease and lack of communication with physicians. Unfortunate childhood experiences may play a role in how an adult
deals with disease. Poor rapport with the physician or lack of detailed
understanding of the nature of asthma may also be factors. It is only
through education that patients may reach a better understanding of the
potential severity and life-threatening aspects of bronchial asthma. Professional counseling may be necessary to reduce denial and to enlighten
patients as to why they often do not follow instructions.

It has been reported recently that patients who have had near-fatal
asthma attacks may have a reduced perception of shortness of breath.

These patients may also have less response to reduced blood oxygen levels. These characteristics would make fatal attacks more likely. By carefully monitoring peak flows these patients stand a better chance of recognizing the increased narrowing of airways that signals an asthma attack. When flows have reduced by 25 percent from the patient's personal best, action must be taken at once. Written instructions help ensure an appropriate response.

Who Is Most Likely to Experience a Near-Fatal Attack?

Patients who have already experienced a severe attack that required respiratory support are the likeliest candidates for fatal asthmatic attacks. When respiratory support is needed the patient's airway or windpipe is intubated with a tube connected to a mechanical ventilator or respirator. Another characteristic that identifies "high risk" patients is an extremely variable or unstable airflow. These patients may have peak flows that drop or increase precipitously. Patients who have required frequent courses of oral corticosteroids or who are maintained on oral steroids should also be considered at greater risk for severe attacks.

About 10–25 percent of all deaths from asthma occur within three hours after the onset of an attack. These patients may progress from minimal symptoms to a collapse of their respirations in a short time. Investigators term this malady "sudden asphyxic asthma." For most patients there is a longer period during which the patient and physician can detect deterioration and instability and act quickly to avoid severe and near-fatal episodes. Without careful home monitoring of peak flows and close communication and compliance with physician instructions, patients who are at high risk for severe asthmatic attacks are likely to experience repeated episodes.

A Case of Fatal Asthma

Several years ago I received a message to call a New York City policeman about the discovery of the body of a 66-year-old woman who had been under my care for asthma. The patrolman had been called by neighbors to enter the patient's apartment since she was not answering her door or phone. A number of people had seen her enter her building in some distress. She had used her bronchodilator spray in the lobby of her building and had not been seen or heard from since. When the policeman and neighbors entered the apartment they found my patient in a chair, still in her overcoat, clutching her bronchodilator spray. The patient had apparently died soon after entering her apartment.

This patient was a delightful woman who edited a foreign policy journal. Office visits were often forums for discussion of a number of topics and she enjoyed debating different points of view. Unfortunately, she had severe asthma that required frequent courses of corticosteroid as well as a long list of other medications. I had seen her about a month before she died, noted significant wheezing and prescribed oral corticosteroids. She was afraid of further steroid use and resisted. "I can just use my asthma spray a little more and I'll be alright." Further discussion revealed she had stopped or reduced a number of her medicines on her own ("I don't think I need them").

Fatal asthma is always tragic since it can usually be prevented. I often wonder what the outcome would have been if this patient had taken her prescribed medication. A number of physicians have said "no one should die of asthma." Unfortunately, these deaths still occur.

Support Systems

Adult Asthma

In managing bronchial asthma it helps the patient to have a support system, particularly helpful for patients with moderate or severe asthma who may need emergency care. For adults this should include a "care partner" who is aware of the patient's illness, physician name and phone number, pharmacy number and who has access to a list of the patient's medications as well as the written instructions that the patient has received from the physician. The patient as well as the care partner should know the location of the nearest emergency room in case of a severe attack. Patients should choose carefully their care partner in terms of proximity and accessibility.

A support group may also be helpful for patients with bronchial asthma. Patients with asthma may have experienced severe attacks and have fears concerning future episodes and dependency on medication. In addition patients may fear to exercise and undertake social activities. Many patients may have been misinformed as to the nature of their illness ("it's all in your head") and have been objects of ridicule. Patients should look to their local lung association or medical society if their physician is not familiar with a specific program. These support groups should be managed by a physician who is a specialist in respiratory diseases. As noted, the primary source of information should be the patient's physician but a support group may further the patient's knowledge and ability to cope with this disease. Patients who have difficult problems in these areas may benefit from professional counseling. The primary physician should be the source of a referral.

Childhood Asthma

In children with bronchial asthma parents usually serve as the care partner. It is extremely important that all members of the child's family be aware of the nature of this disease as well as of the treatment needed. Conflicts can be avoided through proper education directed by the child's physician. This education should also be directed to teachers and friends who are involved in the child's daily activities.

Children may have problems accepting that they have an illness that may cause restrictions on their activities. They may suffer embarrassment at school or play when they suffer attacks. The physician and parent must reinforce a positive attitude in the child regarding asthma to avoid loss of self-esteem and development of poor self-image. Emphasis should be made on maintaining as close to normal activities at home and school including exercise. This should be understood by teachers as well as parents. The school nurse or physician should be made aware of the child's illness and should have on record the child's physician's name and a list of the child's medications.

Asthma Camps

Support groups for children and parents are available that take the form of "asthma camps" or year-round activities. The physician should be able to direct or advise parents in contacting these groups. See appendix A for a list of national organizations that can provide names of these groups.

Stress and Asthma

Asthma has often been associated with anxiety and stress to such an extent that many individuals have erroneously attributed the disease to a psychological disorder. A recent study has documented that anxiety occurs no more frequently in patients with bronchial asthma than in the general population. The same appears true for depression.

Anxiety and Depression

In the more severe asthmatic the level of anxiety increases, usually due to feelings of breathlessness and chest tightness experienced more frequently by patients with moderate to severe asthma. Patients who have suffered severe attacks and may have had emergency care or hospitalization may also suffer increased anxiety. Depression may also develop in a setting of chronic bronchial asthma as with any other chronic illness.

Although anxiety and depression may occur in patients with bronchial asthma there is no evidence they cause the disease. It is likely, however, that they are aggravating factors in the course of this illness. Therefore, every effort should be made to reduce your stress and to treat anxiety and depression. This is accomplished best by psychological counseling. Relaxation techniques and biofeedback have also been helpful in reducing stress in patients with bronchial asthma. As a rule tranquilizers should be avoided since they may affect your respiratory drive and decrease your awareness of shortness of breath. Some antidepressants may also have adverse effects on the respiratory system. Before any medication is prescribed for anxiety and/or depression there must be close consultation between the primary physician and the consulting psychiatrist.

The Asthma Diet

Patients with bronchial asthma can also participate in their care and management by carefully monitoring their diet. Although there is no extensive evidence that ingestion of a certain food product is beneficial in treatment of asthma there is evidence that sensitive asthmatics should avoid certain foods, preservatives, and dyes.

Patients who have experienced allergic reactions to specific foods must carefully avoid these products. Immediate reactions may include development of hives (urticaria), wheezing, collapse of the circulation and swelling of the throat (anaphylaxis). Common sources of allergic or asthmatic reactions include shrimp and other shellfish, eggs, milk, soy, and peanuts. Asthma attacks triggered by food allergies are much more common in children, particularly those with the allergic skin rash known as eczema. In adults these reactions are much less frequent and do not often trigger asthmatic attacks.

It is important to distinguish between a history of a specific allergic reaction that a patient has experienced and a positive allergy test alone. In many instances a positive allergy test (skin or blood) for a particular food may result despite the fact that the patient has ingested the food without reaction. In patients who have severe, unstable asthma it may be helpful to withdraw this food or food group and observe the patient's response. This should not be necessary in patients with less severe asthma that is well controlled.

A recent study has suggested that a diet rich in magnesium may be beneficial to lung function and may actually reduce wheezing and bronchial irritability. Magnesium is found in cereals, nuts, green vegetables, and dairy products. In patients who are not sensitive to these products, a diet rich in magnesium may help.

Sulfites

Sulfites are a common food and beverage preservative that may cause asthmatic attacks in sensitive individuals. These preservatives have been used to make products appear "fresh" and reduce spoilage. Salad bars in restaurants were common sources of sulfite exposure until 1986 when the FDA banned the use of sulfites on fruits and vegetables served as "fresh." It is believed that the irritant producing the asthmatic reaction is sulfur dioxide gas liberated from salts of sulfite, bisulfite or metabisulfite.

Not all asthmatics are sensitive to sulfites. As a rule, however, it is best for all asthmatics to avoid sulfites, especially if they have had asthmatic reactions while dining in restaurants ("restaurant asthma"). Patients who are sensitive will have immediate asthmatic reactions. Some of the products containing sulfites that may cause reactions include processed potatoes, baked products, fresh shrimp, fruit drinks, dried fruits, beer, and wine. Some domestic wines are now labeled if they contain sulfites.

Sulfites have been used as preservatives in medications, too, including some asthma medications. Some nebulizer solutions may contain sulfites. This would explain why some patients may experience bronchospasm instead of bronchodilatation after a nebulizer treatment. For these sulfite-sensitive patients nebulizer solutions that do not contain sulfites are available.

Tartrazine

Tartrazine, a yellow dye (FD&C Yellow Dye #5) that has been used in foods (i.e. margarine) and medications has been demonstrated to cause asthmatic attacks in certain sensitive individuals. At this time it appears this is a rare reaction affecting only a few patients. Those who have experienced attacks after ingestion of tartrazine should avoid it and check carefully for the presence of this substance in foods and medications.

Do I Have to Change My Job?

When considering how an occupation impacts on bronchial asthma you must consider several factors. The environment may have a substantial influence on asthma. Working outdoors in cold air may trigger asthmatic attacks. High degrees of air pollution with exposure to ozone, sulfur dioxide, and particulates may affect asthmatic workers with outdoor jobs. Patients with known allergies to pollens and mold spores as well as other allergens may have to work in air-conditioned environments.

Occupational asthma will be discussed in chapter 8. This condition is created by a work exposure and must be distinguished from the worsening of a preexisting condition in the workplace. It is clear that allergic individuals may be likelier to develop occupational asthma. Asthmatic patients should research their occupations for the incidence of work-related illnesses.

Since asthma may worsen with exercise it is important for a patient to consider how much exertion is required by a particular occupation. Heavy exertion may have to be avoided to reduce the incidence of asthma attacks. Just as the athlete may benefit from premedication with a B_2-agonist or cromolyn sodium before exercise, the worker may also use this approach if high degrees of exertion are required.

With the above precautions and adjustments it should be possible to avoid changing a patient's occupation due to the presence of bronchial asthma.

Achieving Your Asthma Goals

One of the treatment goals of bronchial asthma is achieving a lifestyle as normal as you can. Patients who actively participate in their care will often achieve this goal. As noted previously, participation includes self-monitoring and education, avoidance and elimination of irritating substances from your environment, adjustment of activity and diet, and communication with the physician. These steps require time and effort but the benefits of improvement will certainly be forthcoming.

CHAPTER 7

Asthma and Pregnancy

ASTHMA complicates from 4–6 percent of all pregnancies and is considered one of the common problems that may occur during pregnancy. It may also be a serious complication of pregnancy that affects both mother and child.

Rationale for Treatment

Treating asthma during pregnancy varies little from the general treatment of bronchial asthma. The basis of this principle is that the developing fetus depends on the maternal circulation for its supply of oxygen. If the mother suffers uncontrolled asthma, oxygen levels are reduced, creating a threat to the unborn child. Therefore, the medications for treating asthma are usually maintained during pregnancy. Any medication judged unnecessary or which is unsafe during pregnancy should be withdrawn.

Complications of Unstable Asthma and Pregnancy

Studies have shown that pregnant women with uncontrolled, unstable asthma have complicated pregnancies. These complications include premature birth, increased perinatal mortality, and low birth weight. Pregnant women with severe asthma may suffer from high blood pressure, vaginal hemorrhage, toxemia, and have induced or complicated labor.

Fetal Monitoring

Once pregnancy is confirmed, a patient's obstetrician and the physician responsible for the treatment of the patient's asthma should confer. In view of the potential for complications during pregnancy, fetal monitoring will be stressed. In women with moderate or severe asthma this monitoring will include early ultrasonography (twelve to twenty weeks). In these patients and those who have had frequent asthma attacks during pregnancy, this procedure and monitoring of the fetal heart rate will be repeated frequently during the third trimester.

Diagnosing Asthma During Pregnancy

Asthma may occur for the first time during pregnancy. The diagnosis may be obscured because shortness of breath is common in pregnancy. Increased progesterone levels in pregnancy seem to stimulate respiration resulting in hyperventilation and shortness of breath. This may occur early in pregnancy. In the later stages of pregnancy shortness of breath is also common due to enlargement of the uterus limiting full inspiration. Asthma may still be diagnosed correctly, however, with a thorough history and physical exam combined with spirometry. Flow rate measurements remain accurate in pregnancy even in the third trimester when lung volumes may be reduced by enlargement of the uterus. Oxygen measurements are particularly useful in monitoring asthma during pregnancy. This may be done easily with the pulse oximeter. Any significant decrease in oxygen levels must be closely followed and reversed through aggressive treatment.

Course of Asthma During Pregnancy

The course of asthma during pregnancy has been the subject of study. Just as the disease varies from patient to patient, the severity of asthma during pregnancy will also vary. Approximately a third of patients will suffer worsening of their symptoms while the rest will improve or stay the same. This course also appears to be consistent for subsequent pregnancies. If asthma worsens it often happens between twenty-four and thirty-six weeks of the pregnancy with subsequent improvement. Exacerbations during labor and delivery are rare. Approximately three months post-partum patients will usually return to the degree of asthma they were experiencing prior to pregnancy.

Asthma Medications During Pregnancy

The general principles of maintaining good control of bronchial asthma should be vigorously applied throughout a patient's pregnancy. Patients should maintain their environmental control precautions and avoid as many allergens as possible (see chapter 6). Peak flows should be recorded daily and medications maintained and adjusted accordingly. Understandably, there is a natural reluctance to take medications during pregnancy. In general, asthma medications have been found to be safe during pregnancy and should be continued under guidance of the physician in consultation with the patient's obstetrician.

General Guidelines: Preferred Medications

The data on the effects of the asthma drugs during pregnancy comes from both human and animal studies. The results of animal studies should be reviewed with the knowledge that effects noted in animals may not apply to humans. Some general guidelines for use of asthma drugs can be applied. Inhaled medications should be preferred since these agents do not have as much total body effect as oral or injectable agents. As a rule, medications that have been in use longer should also be preferred since there is greater experience with their use.

Which Drugs Are Preferred During Pregnancy?

Bronchodilators
B_2-AGONISTS The inhaled B_2-agonists (albuterol, metaproterenol, pirbuterol, terbutaline) are the first-line bronchodilators for as-needed use

during pregnancy. As a group, there is extensive human experience with no evidence of fetal injury. Animal studies are also generally without evidence for adverse effects except at high doses. Terbutaline has often been preferred due to negative animal studies. When given by inhalation in normal dosages all the above agents may be used safely throughout pregnancy, labor, and delivery. The B_2-agonists may also be used orally and by nebulization if deemed necessary. If a B-agonist is given by mouth, terbutaline would be considered the preferred oral agent. In patients with mild asthma (no more than two attacks a week; no nocturnal attacks), the B_2-agonists may be adequate for controlling the patient's bronchial asthma during pregnancy.

AVOID NON-SELECTIVE AGENTS Non-selective B-agonists are best avoided during pregnancy. These agents, such as epinephrine (adrenaline) and isoproterenol have both beta-1 and beta-2 effects. Animal studies of these agents have demonstrated abnormal embryo development. Reports from human studies have raised questions concerning their safety. In view of the fact that the selective B_2-agonists are available there is no need to utilize the non-selective medications.

THEOPHYLLINE Theophylline may also be used as a bronchodilator in pregnancy. There is extensive favorable human experience with this agent. Theophylline may be used intravenously as aminophylline in an emergency. It is essential that blood levels be monitored closely during pregnancy. It is recommended that theophylline levels should not be greater than 12 mg/L since infants born of women with higher levels have been found to have adverse effects of theophylline such as jitteriness, vomiting, and rapid heart beat.

ANTI-CHOLINERGIC AGENTS The anti-cholinergic agent ipratropium bromide has not been studied in humans during pregnancy. Animal studies, however, have not shown any evidence of abnormal fetal development. Since this agent is a relatively weak bronchodilator in asthmatic patients, it should not be considered a preferred agent during pregnancy.

Anti-Inflammatory Agents

CROMOLYN SODIUM   Cromolyn sodium is a nonsteroidal anti-inflammatory agent that may be used safely during pregnancy. Both human and animal studies have resulted in favorable results. In view of the extremely low incidence of adverse effects of cromolyn sodium, it should be regarded as the preferred anti-inflammatory agent in pregnancy. In patients for whom cromolyn is not effective, the inhaled corticosteroids should be introduced. Both agents may be given in patients with severe bronchial asthma.

INHALED CORTICOSTEROIDS: BECLOMETHASONE   Anti-inflammatory agents are also needed during pregnancy for patients with more than mild asthma. Inhaled corticosteroids are effective agents that can be used safely during pregnancy. Of the agents available in the United States the greatest human experience has been with beclomethasone. The results have been extremely favorable making beclomethasone the preferred agent. Triamcinolone and flunisolide have not been studied in humans although animal studies are favorable.

SYSTEMIC CORTICOSTEROIDS   Systemic corticosteroids (oral and injectable) may also be needed to treat severe asthma attacks during pregnancy. These agents may be used safely and should not be withheld due to fear of adverse effects on a patient's pregnancy. Human studies have shown only a slight increase in low birth weight and premature births in patients receiving systemic corticosteroids for prolonged periods throughout pregnancy. There has been no evidence of increased birth defects secondary to the use of corticosteroids during pregnancy in large human studies.

NEDOCROMIL SODIUM   Nedocromil sodium resembles cromolyn and is another non-steroidal anti-inflammatory. At this time there is no human experience to refer to although animal studies are favorable. For this reason, cromolyn sodium would be the preferred alternative to inhaled corticosteroids.

Medications for Related Conditions During Pregnancy

Allergic Rhinitis and Sinusitis

There is a high incidence of allergic rhinitis and sinusitis in patients with bronchial asthma. There is a greater frequency of sinusitis during pregnancy. Upper and lower respiratory tract infections, including pneumonia may occur during pregnancy. Treatment of these conditions should not be delayed since they may trigger more severe asthma attacks. Many medications can be used safely for these conditions while some should definitely be avoided.

Intranasal Sprays

Allergic rhinitis like hay fever may be treated with intranasal topical corticosteroid sprays as well as intranasal cromolyn sodium. Of the intranasal steroids, beclomethasone is the preferred agent due to its large human experience. The aerosol spray treatments are preferred over oral antihistamines.

Antibiotics

Antibiotics may be needed during pregnancy to treat specific infections. Indiscriminate use of antibiotics should be avoided especially when viral infection is most likely as in the common cold. Tetracycline, sulfonamides (in late pregnancy), and the quinalones should be avoided during pregnancy. Penicillin and its derivatives such as amoxicillin may be used safely. For penicillin allergic patients erythromycin may be substituted. Sulfonamides may be used in early or midpregnancy.

Antihistamines

Antihistamines like chlorpheniramine and tripelennamine may be used safely during pregnancy in patients unresponsive to the topical sprays. One adverse effect of these antihistamines is drowsiness. The newer non-sedating antihistamines like terfenadine, loratadine, and astemizole have not been studied in humans during pregnancy.

Decongestants

Decongestants may be indicated to relieve persistent and severe nasal symptoms in rhinitis and the common cold. Human experience with pseudoephredrine has been favorable although animal studies have shown fetal abnormalities. An alternative is oxymetazoline nasal spray or drops for a period not to exceed five days. One drawback to oxymetazoline is a patient's tendency to become dependent on its decongestant effect from prolonged use.

Expectorants

Expectorant may be prescribed by the physician to help loosen thick secretions. Iodides, a common ingredient in expectorants, should be avoided during pregnancy and are being withdrawn by the FDA. Guaifenesin may be used safely during pregnancy to help mobilize secretions. Severe cough from lower respiratory tract infections may be harmful and traumatic. A cough suppressant, dextromethorphan, has been used with favorable results during pregnancy. It should be noted, however, that cough may serve a useful purpose in clearing mucus and in many instances should not be suppressed. Cough may also signal that asthma has become more severe. This should be acknowledged by reviewing the patient's history and physical in conjunction with airflow measurements. It is vital to be aware of the ingredients in any cough mixture. Many preparations contain several medications including antihistamines, alcohol, and aspirin which should be avoided by most individuals with asthma.

The Common Cold

Some simple measures can help treat the common cold. A buffered saline nasal spray can moisturize irritated nasal membranes and flush dried mucus. Patients should force fluids; warm fluids provide some relief from nasal congestion. Bedrest can also help and often shortens recovery. For severe symptoms the decongestants and cough medications noted above can help. All treatment should be directed by the patient's physician. Any persistent fever, sore throat, sinus pain and discharge should prompt quick examination and treatment. Cultures can be obtained to document bacterial infections that will require antibiotic therapy.

In many instances a common cold triggers increased bronchial narrowing, which may occur through throat and bronchial infections as well
as through irritation of the bronchial tubes by postnasal discharge. Peak
flows should be monitored closely during colds to identify when bron-

TABLE 7.   PREFERRED ASTHMA DRUGS DURING PREGNANCY

Bronchodilator

Inhaled B_2-Agonist
Add Theophylline If Needed (Keep Level 8–12 Mg/L)
If Oral B_2-Agonist Needed Use Terbutaline

Anti-Inflammatory Agent

Cromolyn Sodium
Substitute or Add Beclomethasone If No Response
Oral Corticosteroid: Prednisone

For Associated Conditions

Allergic Rhinitis:
Cromolyn Sodium
Beclomethasone
Chlorpheniramine or Tripelennamine (Antihistamines)

Bacterial Infection (Such As Sinusitis):
Amoxicillin (Use Erythromycin If Allergic to Penicillin)

Cough:
Guaifenesin (Expectorant)

choconstriction occurs. Early recognition of bronchial narrowing allows the patient and physician to begin a treatment plan that reverses bronchoconstriction before a severe attack can occur. This plan may include an increase in the number of sprays of a topical corticosteroid or a course of oral steroid.

Labor and Delivery

All of the preferred asthma medications can be continued during labor. In general, patients should continue their normal asthma medications throughout labor. Corticosteroids may also be given in those patients who have been steroid dependent and may have adrenal insufficiency. The type of delivery will be determined by the patient's obstetrician. In patients with severe or unstable asthma, a cesarean section may be necessary.

A 34-year-old woman with severe asthma has been under my care for ten years. Five years ago she asked me if I thought it was medically safe for her to have a child. The patient had been hospitalized for asthma and had required frequent courses of oral corticosteroids. Her daily treatment plan included regular B-agonist, inhaled corticosteroid, cromolyn sodium, and theophylline. We decided to do a detailed pulmonary function test to help in the decision. I knew that she was highly motivated and involved in her care. She was also extremely compliant with her medication routine and called whenever there was a significant drop in her peak flow. I reviewed her breathing tests and found that her lung capacity was 70 percent of normal after she used her bronchodilator spray. The patient's oxygen level was near normal. I told her that I thought she could become pregnant. During her pregnancy she required oral corticosteroids several times and maintained her usual medications. I spoke frequently with her obstetrician. The patient's asthma remained severe but did not worsen and she delivered a healthy baby girl by cesarean section. Her asthma has remained severe and during office visits we sometimes refer to her daughter as the "miracle baby." When I look back at all the factors that had to be considered, I am sure I would make the same decision.

Should Allergy Treatments Be Started or Continued?

Immunotherapy (also called desensitization) has been helpful in reducing asthma attacks in allergic patients although adverse reactions to allergy injections may occur in sensitive individuals. A severe, total body reaction like anaphylaxis would threaten a developing fetus. Anaphylaxis has also been reported to induce labor. For these reasons it is recommended that no allergy treatment or immunotherapy be started during pregnancy.

In patients who have reached maintenance therapy in which dosages of allergens injected are not increased and who are not known to have reactions, immunotherapy may continue as prescribed by the patient's physician. Patients who are extremely sensitive and who have had systemic reactions like anaphylaxis are best not treated.

Is Flu Vaccine Safe During Pregnancy?

A killed vaccine, like influenza vaccine, does not pose a threat during pregnancy. In fact, it is a good idea for patients with moderate to severe asthma to receive influenza vaccine in order to avoid this severe infection that may exacerbate their disease. This vaccine should be administered before December 1st in order to allow enough time for antibody levels to become effective.

After Delivery

Nursing

Asthma medications are commonly found in breast milk but that should not keep asthmatic mothers from breast-feeding. The inhaled medications (B$_2$-agonists, inhaled corticosteroids, cromolyn sodium) do not reach significant levels in breast milk and should have little if any effect on an infant. Oral corticosteroids are secreted in breast milk but only a small fraction of the mother's dosage reaches the infant. Prednisone and prednisolone are also considered compatible with breast-feeding. Theophylline is secreted in breast milk but less than 1 percent of the mother's dose ever reaches the child. In rare instances, excessive irritability has been reported of infants being breast-fed by mothers receiving theophylline. If that occurs and the mother's asthma is well controlled, it is usually possible to interrupt theophylline and adjust other medications.

Avoiding Complications During Pregnancy

To reduce complications that may adversely affect the mother and developing child, asthma should be well-controlled before and during pregnancy. Uncontrolled asthma may reduce oxygen delivery to the fetus and lead to serious complications. Treatment of asthma during pregnancy is similar to the general treatment plan discussed in chapter 5. Most of the asthma medications are clearly safe during pregnancy and should be used normally. Certain medications are preferred and they are listed in this chapter. Unfortunately, their fear of medication side effects during pregnancy has prompted many asthmatic patients to eliminate their medicines, thus increasing their risk of complications. Through patient education and communication with the physician as well as careful use of asthma medications, the risk of complications for pregnant asthmatics can be greatly reduced.

CHAPTER 8

Occupational Asthma

THERE is little doubt that asthma may develop in the workplace, creating a significant health problem. Estimates of the incidence of occupational asthma vary according to the industry. Each year new agents that may cause asthma are identified and another occupation is added to an expanding list. At last count more than 200 agents had been identified as potential causes of occupational asthma.

What Is Occupational Asthma?

Occupational asthma is an illness created in the workplace by a particular material. It is distinguished from preexisting asthma that worsens at work from adverse conditions. Some types of occupational asthma appear to occur more often in allergic individuals, but it is clear that this disease may also occur in nonallergic workers.

The offending agents that produce occupational asthma may occur in many forms, including animal and vegetable proteins, dyes, chemicals, particulates, propellants, and enzymes. These agents can produce reactions in forms such as dusts, vapors, powders, or by direct contact.

Examples of Occupational Asthma

Workers exposed to animals, such as farmers or veterinarians, may develop asthma as a result of sensitization to proteins in animal hair, dander,

TABLE 8. EXAMPLES OF OCCUPATIONAL ASTHMA

Occupation or Industry	Agents
Baker	Flours, Cottonseed Oil
Beautician	Fluorocarbon Propellants, Persulfate
Carpenter, Wood Worker	Wood Dust
Farmer	Soy Bean Dust
Grocery Worker	Plastic Wrapping
Hospital Worker	Latex, Psyllium, Disinfectants
Pesticide Worker	Organophosphates
Pharmaceutical	Antibiotics, Lactose
Plastics, Paint	Toluene Diisocyanate
Postal Workers, Bookbinders	Glue (Fish Origin)
Poultry Workers	Animal Proteins, Aprolium
Printers	Vegetable Gums
Refinery Workers	Platinum Salts, Vanadium
Textile	Cotton, Flax, Hemp Dust
Veterinarians, Laboratory Workers	Animal Dander, Urine
Welder	Stainless Steel Fumes

and urine. Bakers may develop asthma as a result of reactions to flour. Woodworkers may become sensitized to dusts from various woods and develop asthmatic reactions. Workers like butchers who handle plastic wraps may become sensitized to the material. In the plastics and paint industries a substance known as toluene diisocyanate (TDI) has been shown to be particularly sensitizing. Beauticians may develop asthma as a reaction to chemicals and sprays used in their work. Even these few examples of occupational asthma demonstrate how significant this problem may be for workers and industry. A more complete list is in Table 8.

When Should I Suspect I May Have Occupational Asthma?

The basis for such a diagnosis comes from a thorough occupational history linked to physical and laboratory findings under direction of a physician. But the patient is the one who calls medical symptoms to the attention of the physician. A high degree of awareness helps identify what may be occupational sources of asthma.

What to Look for: 'Monday Morning Asthma'

There may be clues that should prompt further investigation. The symptoms of cough, eye irritation, and nasal congestion may occur at work before the wheezing or shortness of breath develops. These symptoms often occur only at work and not in any other environment. The longer a worker is exposed, however, the greater the likelihood of persistent symptoms outside the workplace. "Monday morning asthma" is a term that describes the sudden onset of symptoms when workers return to work. Symptoms may decline somewhat during the week with a great improvement on weekends or during vacations or other absences. Although many reactions are immediate, it is important to recall the late phase of bronchial asthma and how reactions may be delayed and occur hours after leaving the workplace.

Can Occupational Asthma Become Chronic?

Studies have demonstrated that the longer the patient is exposed to the offending agent the more likely the asthma will become chronic. Without information on an individual's occupation (obtained during recording of the patient's medical history) it is easy to see how occupational asthma might be overlooked. Even after a worker leaves a job that has produced occupational asthma, the symptoms may continue for years.

How You Can Help Make the Diagnosis

Patients may be asked by their physician to aid in the diagnosis of occupational asthma. Valuable information can be obtained by using a peak flow meter. Readings of airflows at home and at work may document precipitous drops in the workplace or hours after exposure. This type of "challenge test" is preferred to a laboratory study in which a physician attempts to duplicate workplace conditions.

Obtaining information on other workers who may have developed similar symptoms would also be extremely valuable. The physician may have to contact plant officials or local health authorities to obtain this information. It would be most unusual for occupational asthma to be an isolated occurrence. Screening coworkers may help detect other individuals with early manifestations of occupational asthma.

Treating Occupational Asthma

The best treatment for occupational asthma is ending the patient's exposure to the offending agent. This is particularly important because patients can develop chronic asthma, which is not completely reversible. Asthmatic workers may have to change their occupations.

Options other than leaving a job would be shifting to activities in the same industry that do not involve exposure to the offending agent, as well as protective clothing or filtration masks. Individuals who are trained in a field and who have developed a unique sensitivity may want to consider immunotherapy. This may be especially helpful for those like veterinarians who have become sensitized to animal proteins.

A Growing Problem

The occupational asthma problem is likely to get worse as new offending materials are identified in many industries. This affliction may occur in almost any occupation, always manifested by development of bronchial asthma. The worker often makes the association him or herself between an offending agent and illness. Once an irritating substance is identified, additional occupational asthma cases are usually discovered.

Remember that occupational asthma is a disease that begins in the workplace, so it must be distinguished from preexisting asthma that worsens from work conditions, which might better be called "aggravated asthma." Outside of work, many asthmatics experience attacks with physical exertion. The next chapter discusses the relationship between exercise and asthma.

CHAPTER 9

Exercise and Asthma

A PRIMARY goal of asthma treatment is maintaining as normal a lifestyle for the patient as possible, including exercise. Properly managed patients with asthma should be able to pursue exercise as vigorously as anyone. Some Olympic athletes are asthmatic and have even set world records in their events.

Exercise-Induced Asthma (EIA)

Considerable research has been focused on exercise and asthma. Any asthmatic patient may experience bronchospasm and worsening of their condition after exercise. This response has been termed "exercise-induced asthma (EIA)." In some patients, particularly children with allergic rhinitis, exercise may be the only trigger for asthma, a phenomenon also noted in adults. These patients *only* experience asthma with exercise. EIA probably affects 70–90 percent of asthmatic patients.

How Asthmatics Respond to Exercise

Research has documented that constriction of the bronchial tubes occurs in asthmatics after about five minutes of exercise. Even if the person stops exercising the bronchial tightening may worsen, but after ten to twenty minutes of rest the tubes reopen and airflow returns to the pre-exercise level. If an asthmatic resumes the exercise the degree of constriction may lessen with further activity. Therefore, I recommend that patients with asthma always perform "warm up" exercises followed by a brief rest period before any vigorous exertion.

A Lack of 'Warming'

There is a clear relationship between exercise-induced asthma and warming and humidifying air as it is inhaled. Apparently, asthmatics during exercise do not warm air and add moisture to it in the nasal passages as well as non-asthmatics. When the dryer and cooler air reaches the bronchial tubes it triggers an asthmatic reaction. Any exercise may produce EIA but exercise in cold, dry air produces more intense bronchial spasms. Extremely sensitive asthma patients should avoid exercising in sub-freezing temperatures.

Making the Diagnosis

Research has also shown that exercise-induced asthma may have both an immediate and a late phase. The late phase may occur several hours after the patient has ceased activities. Although a diagnosis of exercise-induced asthma may be evident from a patient's history, doctors may need to perform an exercise test if patients do not manifest asthma any other time. This test is done routinely when performing pulmonary function tests with a bicycle ergometer or a treadmill. Patients may also get valuable information by measuring their peak flows before, during, and after exercise.

How Should Exercise-Induced Asthma Be Treated?

Treating exercise-induced asthma is preventive. Several agents seem to be effective and are easily adapted for both children and adults.

B$_2$-Adrenergic Agonists

The B$_2$-adrenergic agonists are effective in preventing exercise-induced asthma. If a short-acting agent is given ten to fifteen minutes before exertion the immediate bronchoconstriction may be completely blocked. The long-acting B_2-agonists such as salmeterol may be particularly helpful since their lengthy duration may also block the late-phase attack. Remember, however, that long-acting B-agonists take longer to become effective so should be given thirty to forty-five minutes before exercise begins.

B-Agonists for Children

In young children a metered-dose inhaler (MDI) may be difficult to use, so a spacer with or without a facemask may improve medication. Some children, particularly those younger than five, may benefit more from a nebulizer that administers the B-agonist. Another alternative for young children is the oral syrup form of B-agonist taken at least sixty minutes before exercising.

Cromolyn Sodium and Nedocromil Sodium

Cromolyn sodium and nedocromil sodium can also prevent exercise-induced asthma and are an alternative to the B-agonists. In patients with moderate or severe asthma both groups of agents may be used together. Cromolyn and nedocromil can also block the late phase of exercise-induced asthma, but their onset of action may be even slower than the short-acting B-agonists. One study comparing cromolyn and albuterol to prevent exercise-induced asthma, found albuterol more effective.

Theophylline

Theophylline can also prevent exercise-induced asthma but is clearly less effective than the B-agonists, cromolyn, and nedocromil. Inhaled corticosteroids cannot prevent the immediate effects of exercise but their use in asthma maintenance therapy would help prevent late-phase reactions.

Approved Medications

The NCAA and the International Olympic Committee maintain lists of acceptable medications for athletes. Medications approved by the United

States Olympic Committee include B-agonists (aerosol forms only), albuterol, and terbutaline, as well as cromolyn sodium, nedocromil sodium, theophylline, and inhaled corticosteroids.

Guidelines to Follow to Prevent EIA

Some simple guidelines are helpful in preventing exercise-induced asthma. First, do not exercise if you have been experiencing frequent attacks or are still recovering from a recent attack. After an attack, consult your physician before you embark on or resume an exercise program. Second, always pre-medicate with either a B-agonist and/or cromolyn sodium as directed by your physician. Third, always perform warm-up exercises followed by a brief rest before starting your full workout. Fourth, wear a facemask or scarf across your nose and face to warm inspired air if you exercise in the cold. If you experience any difficulty with exercise, tell your physician so you can obtain his or her instructions on adjusting your routine. It would help your physician review your case if you obtain peak flow measurements recorded at the time of distress.

TABLE 9.   HOW TO PREVENT EXERCISE-INDUCED ASTHMA

Avoid Exercise If Your Asthma Is Unstable;
Check with Your Physician If You Are Unsure

Always Perform Warm-Up Exercises;
Rest 5–10 Minutes Before You Begin to Exercise

Use Your Short-Acting B_2-Agonist 15 Minutes Before Exercise
Or a Long-Acting B_2-Agonist 30 Minutes Before Exercise

If You Still Experience Difficulty with Exercise Add to the Above
Cromolyn or Nedocromil Taken One Hour Before Exercise

Avoid Exercise in Extreme Cold (Below Freezing);
Always Wear a Facemask When Exercising in Cold Weather

Avoid Outdoor Exercise When Ozone Levels Are High

How Does Conditioning Affect Asthma?

Recent evidence suggests regular conditioning exercises may have a favorable effect on asthma and the use of medications. Conditioning increases the muscle fitness and improves your body's ability to supply oxygen as fuel. Regular exercise eases breathing effort and increases stamina.

A recent study demonstrated that conditioning of patients with asthma resulted in a greater degree of dilatation of the bronchial tubes after exercise, an effect that reduced their potential for exercise-induced asthma. Clearly, if patients follow these guidelines for preventing exercise-induced asthma, they may benefit greatly from regular exercise.

What Type of Exercise Should I Do?

Almost any form of exercise may be performed by individuals with asthma. Athletes with asthma have distinguished themselves in many diverse competitions including swimming, track and field, cycling, and even cross-country skiing. You should find a form you enjoy and gradually increase your activity.

If you are about to start an exercise program always check first with your physician, who may want you to take an exercise test. Remember, your asthma should be under good control before you start any exercise routine.

You can exercise at home or indoors, especially during the winter months. In fact, indoor exercise may be better for you during high pollen count periods or air pollution alerts. A simple way to begin is with light stretching exercises for the arms, shoulders, and torso. Appendix A lists a workout tape designed especially for asthmatics. Recent research suggests that conditioning the upper body reduces shortness of breath in many patients with chronic respiratory disease. Upper body exercises may include light weights; some asthmatics prefer weight training to more rigorous programs.

Your exercise regimen will succeed best with regular workouts. You do not have to exercise every day. A routine of twenty to thirty minutes of exercise three times a week is good. Many patients vary their exercises for each workout, increasing their conditioning gradually.

Achieving Your Goal of an Active Lifestyle

Asthma does get worse when you exercise, but that fact has not kept individuals with asthma from setting world records in many sports events. Anyone with good control over asthma may begin an exercise program and the conditioning you achieve may help improve your stamina and reduce shortness of breath. Exercise may also help you reduce stress and anxiety as you build confidence and improve your well-being.

This chapter has offered guidelines and suggestions for developing and performing an asthma exercise regimen, whose benefits are clear. The next chapter explores the relationship between asthma and other illnesses that affect the sinuses and the stomach.

CHAPTER 10

Asthma and Related Illnesses

ALTHOUGH asthma is a disease of the lungs it may be influenced by illnesses that affect other parts of the body. In many asthma patients, treating these related illnesses even may improve their bronchial asthma condition. Two common examples are disorders of the nose and sinuses and of the digestive tract. This chapter will discuss the relationship between asthma and these illnesses.

What Are the Sinuses?

The sinuses are a series of bony cavities located in the skull, lined by a surface layer called the epithelium. This thin membrane closely resembles the bronchial tube lining. Each sinus opens into the nasal passages, which have a similar surface lining. Although this thin surface membrane has a pale, innocent appearance it may become severely swollen and produce a copious discharge. Figure 22 shows the location of the sinuses.

The nasal and sinus passages perform several functions vital to healthy breathing including filtering air as it is inhaled, trapping foreign particles and germs, as well as warming and adding moisture to inspired air. The importance of the warming function was highlighted in chapter 9.

Symptoms of Nasal and Sinus Disease

When the lining of the nasal and sinus passages becomes irritated and inflamed the body's response is similar to what occurs in the bronchial tubes during an asthma attack. This reaction may occur in patients with and without allergies. Swelling of this lining creates congestion and stuffiness. In the nose this inflammation is called rhinitis and when inflammation occurs too much mucus may be produced adding to the obstruction. A watery discharge or drip is common with many irritations of the nose and sinuses. Because some of this discharge may be directed back toward the throat it is often termed "post-nasal drip."

In the bony sinuses inhaled germs may take advantage of these wet, warm conditions to produce an infection called sinusitis. When that happens, the back drip may carry disease organisms into the throat and lower respiratory passages. Sinus infections may be slow to resolve and difficult to treat because of lowered blood supply to bony areas. A recent study of

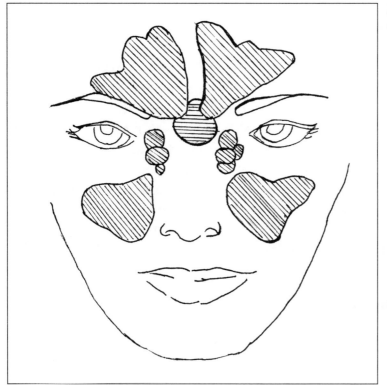

Figure 22.
The Sinuses

sinuses during common colds highlighted the extensive sinus infection and congestion that may exist then. If not adequately treated, sinus disease can become chronic, forming the basis for repeated infections.

How Sinus Disease Can Affect Asthma

Clearly, there is a close relationship between sinus disease and asthma. Patients with active sinus disease may suffer repeated worsening of their asthma. These flare-ups may be partly due to mucus dripping into the throat and windpipe causing cough and irritation. Infection from the sinuses may also be carried into the lower bronchial tree triggering inflammation and asthma. This may often occur at night, another reason for nighttime asthma attacks. Nasal and sinus congestion may also produce obstruction of these passages necessitating mouth-breathing and the absence of warming and moisturizing of inhaled air that the nasal and sinus passages produce may also exacerbate bronchial asthma.

How Is Sinusitis Diagnosed?

The characteristic symptoms of sinus disease include nasal congestion, pain, and a discolored mucus discharge. The pain usually occurs over or near the affected sinus. Often, this pain is felt as a severe headache, particularly over the forehead. Facial swelling is also common and so is tenderness over the affected areas. Examination is commonly done with a flashlight that looks into the nasal passages, often aided by an instrument called a nasal speculum that widens the doctor's field of view into the nose. For a more detailed examination with the ability to better visualize the sinus openings, fiberoptic instruments like the flexible endoscope may be used.

A sinusitis diagnosis may be confirmed by x-ray. Plain sinus films may demonstrate the presence of fluid in the sinus cavities or a thickening of the lining. The more highly detailed CAT scan (computerized axial tomography) is now widely used to diagnose sinusitis because it may pick up disease plain x-ray films miss.

Treating Rhinitis and Sinusitis

Antibiotics

The primary treatment for acute sinusitis is antibiotics for eradicating infection. A prolonged course is often needed because the blood supply is limited to bony areas like the sinuses. This course may vary but a typical treatment takes three weeks.

Establishing Drainage

In sinus disease it is crucial to establish good drainage, which is often achieved with decongestants like pseudoephedrine. Antihistamines can also help, particularly in allergic patients but may not be a good idea for many asthmatics owing to the risk of drying up the bronchial secretion. To avoid excessive dryness, decongestants are often combined with an expectorant like guaifenesin. A saline nasal spray may help rinse out dried secretions and add moisture to dry membranes.

Treating Chronic Sinusitis

Even after a sinus infection has been eradicated, many patients will continue to experience congestion, pain, and recurring bouts of sinus infection. In patients with chronic disease, particularly allergic ones, adding intranasal corticosteroid sprays may be extremely helpful in reducing inflammation. Beclomethasone, budesonide, fluticasone, flunisolide, and triamcinolone are available in the United States. Intranasal cromolyn sodium may also help these patients. An intranasal preparation of nedocromil sodium should be available soon.

Should You Consider Surgery?

In patients who suffer from persistent sinus infections despite courses of appropriate antibiotics, a surgical drainage procedure may be needed. A sinus CAT scan documenting the presence of infection and maximal medical therapy should have been given before surgery. When possible, this surgery is increasingly performed through the endoscope. The technique is less traumatic than older sinus drainage procedures and is often performed in an outpatient setting.

Physicians must individualize treatment of sinus disease for each patient. Aggressive treatment of sinus disease, however, may also improve the control of bronchial asthma.

Treating Rhinitis

Treating rhinitis in many ways is similar to sinusitis. Decongestants and antihistamines may be prescribed for patients with bronchial asthma who do not experience the adverse excessive dryness and "plugging" of the bronchial tubes. A saline nasal mist can help provide moisture to the nasal lining. Intranasal topical corticosteroid sprays (beclomethasone, budesonide, triamcinolone, flunisolide, fluticasone) and cromolyn sodium are extremely helpful in treating rhinitis. These agents do not produce excessive dryness and may be preferred over decongestants and antihistamines. Adverse effects of topical corticosteroid nasal sprays include minor irritation or stinging and, rarely, bleeding from the nasal lining.

What Are Nasal Polyps?

Nasal polyps are fleshy growths or extensions of the nasal and sinus lining. They are common in patients with bronchial asthma and may occur with or without allergy. They often occur in patients older than forty who are not allergic but who have severe rhinitis. Common symptoms are constant nasal stuffiness as well as a loss or reduction of the senses of smell and/or taste.

The importance of nasal polyps is related to their ability to block the nasal and sinus passages, which may also be the source of poor drainage of sinuses that leads to recurring sinus infections. The presence of nasal polyps in adult patients who are not allergic often identifies a more severe group of asthmatics. This group also has a greater hypersensitivity to aspirin and related medications (see chapter 13).

Treating Nasal Polyps

Administering topical intranasal corticosteroid sprays often helps. Oral corticosteroids may be used to shrink polyps in patients with severe disease. In those who do not respond and who have severe obstructions, polypectomy should be considered. When feasible, this procedure is also being performed endoscopically. Before polypectomy occurs, the patient's asthma must be under good control, which may demand pre-treatment with oral corticosteroids. Unfortunately, polyps tend to recur.

Asthma and the Stomach

More and more clearly there seems to be some relationship between bronchial asthma and stomach function. Asthmatics often suffer from digestive problems, frequently complaining about excess stomach acid. Treating stomach disorders may actually improve the control of unstable asthmatics who are prone to frequent attacks.

The Esophagus

Every human digestive tract includes a feeding passage known as the esophagus through which food passes before entering the stomach to begin digestion. The esophagus is in the chest just behind the windpipe and starts at about the same level as the voice box (larynx). At the lower end of the esophagus a muscular ring or sphincter that relaxes to open and tightens to close ensures stomach contents remain in the stomach where they are exposed to acid. In many digestive disorders the esophageal sphincter may malfunction allowing a reflux of acid back into the esophagus. This is called gastroesophageal reflux disease (GERD).

Increasing evidence suggests this disorder is related to reduced motion or motility of the feeding passage and stomach. An associated condition is overproduction of acid or hyperacidity. A common contributing condition to GERD is a hiatal hernia where a fold of the stomach lining protrudes upward into the esophagus.

Asthma and Reflux

Research shows a high incidence of gastroesophageal reflux in patients with bronchial asthma. It is unclear how much of a contributing factor GERD is to bronchial asthma since many studies have resulted in conflicting conclusions. Also unclear is how acid reflux aggravates bronchial asthma. In rare cases the actual aspiration of acid into the bronchial tubes may occur producing severe inflammation. Merely the presence of acid in the esophagus may even trigger a reflex leading to bronchoconstriction. Despite these controversies, some patients with GERD and asthma have benefited from the treatment of reflux which has reduced the frequency of their asthma attacks.

Medications That May Aggravate Stomach Disorders

Several asthma medications may irritate your stomach. Theophylline may irritate the stomach lining: gastritis. In patients with preexisting hyperacidity, theophylline may aggravate their condition and increase reflux. Oral corticosteroids may produce gastritis as well as ulceration of the stomach lining.

When Should You Suspect Gastroesophageal Reflux?

The symptoms of gastroesophageal reflux are obvious, including heartburn and belching, complaints most apparent after meals and during the hours of sleep when an asthma patient is reclining. Examining the voice box may reveal signs of acid irritation. Further proof of reflux may be obtained through endoscopic examination of the esophagus as well as through x-rays of the upper digestive tract. Asthma attacks often occur at night, so it may be unclear whether an attack is related to reflux. A distinguishing feature of GER-related asthma may be the patient's inability to prevent nighttime attacks despite maximal therapy.

Treating Gastroesophageal Reflux

Patients may reduce reflux by not eating at least two hours before bedtime and by elevating the head of their bed by six to eight inches. Patients should avoid alcohol, caffeine, and highly seasoned foods. Medications like theophylline and oral corticosteroids may need to be reduced or eliminated in patients who do not respond to medical measures for controlling reflux.

Many medications can be used to treat reflux. These medications should only be directed by your physician. Too many patients overuse antacids trying to reduce heartburn. Your physician may prescribe one of a group of medications called H-2 antagonists (cimetadine, ranitidine, famotidine, nizatidine, omeprazole) that inhibit acid production in patients with gastroesophageal reflux. Studies of patients with asthma and reflux who were treated with omeprazole have shown improvment in the asthmatic condition.

Your physician may also prescribe a medication that increases esophagus motility and emptying of the stomach, thus reducing reflux. These medications are called prokinetic agents and are taken before meals and at bedtime. Metoclopramide was the first prokinetic agent introduced in the United States, but was found to have significant adverse effects such as drowsiness. A second-generation prokinetic, cisapride, has an extremely low incidence of adverse effects and has effectively reduced GERD. In rare instances medical therapy may fail and surgical treatment should be considered.

Aggressively treating gastroesophageal reflux in patients with uncontrolled asthma may successfully reduce the frequency of asthma attacks. This condition should be searched out in patients whose asthma is difficult to control despite maximal therapy.

Conclusion: Look for Related Illnesses

In this chapter asthma and illnesses that may affect the nose and sinuses and digestive tract have been considered. Patients who have unstable asthma should look outside their chests to spot aggravating factors like sinusitis and reflux of stomach acid. In many patients identifying and treating these related illnesses may improve their bronchial asthma condition.

Asthma and Special Considerations

Asthma and Surgery

SURGERY may present several problems for asthmatics and must be approached carefully. To avoid complications there should be close communication prior to the procedure between the surgeon and the physician responsible for managing the patient's asthma.

Possible Complications

Complications may arise from several sources in patients with asthma who undergo surgery. When general anesthesia is required, the windpipe is intubated with a tube connected to a respirator. Under anesthesia, the respirator provides mechanical breathing and ensures the exchange of oxygen and carbon dioxide. In asthma patients, intubating the windpipe may trigger reflexes originating in the throat that can lead to bronchoconstriction. Therefore, alternatives to general anesthesia—local, regional, and spinal—should always be considered, depending greatly upon the type of surgery and the surgeon's preference.

Further complications may be caused by bronchoconstriction during and after surgery. Oxygen and carbon dioxide levels may be affected. Surgery is often a source of decreased depth of breathing; as a result the small air sacs of the lung may collapse, a condition known as atelectasis. This condition may also lower oxygen levels and combined with the presence of bronchoconstriction can produce an even greater drop in blood oxygen. More severe atelectasis can be expected in patients who undergo general anesthesia. Thick bronchial mucus of asthma may clog airways and increase the risk of lung infection.

Complications vary greatly depending on the surgery performed. The greatest risk occurs from procedures involving the chest such as heart or lung operations. Surgery performed on the upper abdomen, such as gall bladder removal, may also impact lung function significantly.

How to Avoid Complications from Surgery

The Preoperative Evaluation

If surgery is needed, a preoperative evaluation should be performed by the primary physician, even in patients who are under good control because complications may arise in any asthmatic patient. Patients with moderate to severe asthma are certainly at greater risk for complications and should have diligent preoperative checkups.

During evaluation the patient's history, medications, and flow rates or spirometry should be reviewed. The frequency of asthma attacks should be noted as well as the person's need for bronchodilator sprays and corticosteroids.

Allergies to medications and previous reactions to anesthesia should be noted at this time. The patient should be instructed on how to take asthma medication before surgery since many procedures are now performed outpatient or the same day.

When Surgery Should Be Postponed

Patients who undergo elective surgery who are not under good control should postpone their procedures to allow proper administration of medication. In emergencies, this delay may not be possible, so asthma therapy may have to be given intravenously during and after surgery.

Preparing for Surgery

Preparing for surgery may include a course of oral corticosteroids in patients who are symptomatic or show significant reductions in flow rates on spirometry. In stable patients the medication regimen should continue right up to the time of surgery. To avoid reflex bronchoconstriction, B$_2$-agonists may be given by inhalation just before surgery. Because all oral intake is usually stopped for several hours before surgery, patients receiving theophylline may be affected, although long-acting preparations may maintain blood levels for up to twelve hours. In patients who must maintain a therapeutic blood level for good control of their asthma, intravenous aminophylline may ensure a constant level.

Patients with moderate to severe asthma who have required daily doses or frequent courses of oral corticosteroids should receive intravenous injections of corticosteroids at the time of surgery to prevent exacerbation of their condition and possible adrenal insufficiency. Steroids should also be given in the postoperative period. Inhalation therapy with bronchodilators like B-agonists and anticholinergic medication should also be continued after surgery.

After Surgery

Once the asthma patient has stabilized after surgery, an attempt should be made to resume the patient's maintenance asthma medication as soon as possible. In patients whose asthma has worsened, an oral steroid course may be given with gradual lowering of dosage.

With careful preparation that identifies patients at greater risk, surgery complications can be avoided. Newer anesthesia techniques that avoid intubation may also prevent serious complications. Even in the mildest asthmatic patient preparation is needed before surgery.

Aspirin Hypersensitivity and Asthma

Allergy to aspirin and related medications may trigger asthmatic attacks in as many as 20 percent of adult asthmatics. This sensitivity appears to be more common in severe adult asthmatics, especially those who have nasal polyps and sinusitis. These patients are also often steroid dependent. However, this reaction may occur in any asthmatic patient although it is rare in children. The cause of this reaction appears to be related to inhibition by aspirin of the enzyme cyclooxygenase. A large group of medications that also produce this inhibition, the nonsteroidal anti-inflammatory drugs (NSAIDs), may also cause the same asthmatic reaction.

Characteristic Features of Aspirin-Sensitive Asthma

The most common presentation is an adult patient who first develops severe nasal symptoms of congestion and drip. Sinusitis may also develop and nasal polyps are often discovered on examination. In these patients, bronchial asthma may not be present at first but tends to develop after the nasal problems. Once asthma surfaces, it is often severe and unstable.

Several characteristics of aspirin-hypersensitivity asthma should be emphasized. Aspirin may produce an asthmatic attack even in patients who have previously taken it without any reaction. These attacks are usually severe, occurring within one hour of aspirin ingestion. The reaction may include flushing, nasal congestion, eye irritation in addition to the asthmatic attack. Even a single aspirin tablet (or other anti-inflammatory agent that may cause bronchoconstriction) may produce a potentially fatal asthma attack. Once sensitivity to aspirin is established it does not resolve and asthma patients should never again take this medication.

How the Diagnosis Is Made

The definitive diagnosis of aspirin-hypersensitivity asthma may only be made by documenting a reaction to this medication. A challenge test may be performed by experienced physicians with immediate access to medication to counter a severe reaction. Documentation may also be made through an accurate medical history. If so, the physician may not feel a challenge test is needed. Because of the danger of developing a severe asthma attack from aspirin ingestion, all asthma patients should avoid using aspirin.

TABLE 10.	MEDICATIONS THAT MAY PRODUCE ASTHMA IN ASPIRIN-SENSITIVE PATIENTS*
Drug Name	Brand Name
Aspirin	Empirin, Fiorinal, Percodan, Equagesic, Ecotrin**
Diclofenac	Voltaren
Diflunisal	Dolobid
Fenoprofen	Nalfon
Ketoprofen	Orudis
Flurbiprofen	Ansaid
Ibuprofen	Advil, Motrin, Nuprin
Indomethacin	Indocin
Mefenamic Acid	Ponstel
Naproxen	Aleve, Anaprox, Naprosyn
Piroxicam	Feldene
Sulfinpyrazone	Anturane
Sulindac	Clinoril
Tolmetin	Tolectin
Oxaprozin	Daypro

*This is only a partial list. New NSAIDs are being introduced.

**Also a partial list. Many O-T-C medications contain aspirin and are not listed.

Nonsteroidal Anti-Inflammatory Drugs (NSAIDs)

Nonsteroidal anti-inflammatory drugs (NSAIDs) that also inhibit the enzyme cyclooxygenase may also cause a severe asthma reaction. For a partial list of these drugs see Table 10. Many new NSAIDs are being introduced that are widely prescribed for pain, headache, joint disease, and menstrual cramps. Two NSAIDs, ibuprofen and naproxen, are available without prescription. Aspirin and ibuprofen are often included in "cold remedies" sold over the counter. Patients should carefully review the ingredients of any O-T-C medication and if unsure of its safely, consult their physician. Generally, you should avoid "cold pills" since they often combine aspirin and antihistamines, two agents that may produce adverse reactions in patients with bronchial asthma.

Because of possible asthmatic reactions to NSAIDs, patients with asthma should avoid these medications. In patients with illnesses such as rheumatoid arthritis where these medications are often needed, anti-inflammatory medications that do not inhibit cyclooxygenase may be tried. If a NSAIDs that may produce asthma must be given, it is best to administer the first dose in the physician's office with emergency medication for asthma on hand. Another approach in patients who may need a NSAID and who have asthma is to try and "desensitize" them to the medication, a procedure that would likely require hospitalization for close observation.

Alternatives to aspirin and NSAIDs include acetaminophen, sodium thiosalicylate and choline magnesium trisalicylate. Acetaminophen, widely available without prescription, has reportedly produced asthma attacks in a small number of patients. This reaction is extremely rare and as a rule, this drug represents a safe alternative to aspirin and the NSAIDs. Sodium thiosalicylate and choline magnesium trisalicylate are anti-inflammatory drugs that do not inhibit cyclooxygenase and are safe alternatives to aspirin and NSAIDs. These medications are only available by prescription.

Nocturnal Asthma

Nighttime can be an extremely difficult period for individuals with bronchial asthma. All asthma patients have more sensitive airways at night. Those with increased attacks at night, "nocturnal asthma," have been found to experience an eightfold increase in airway hyperreactivity. Remember, the presence of nocturnal attacks is one of the factors that differentiates mild from moderate and severe asthmatics.

Adding to the significance of nocturnal asthma is increasing data that fatal attacks are more common at night. Several studies show a greater incidence of severe and fatal attacks between midnight and eight A.M. This data has prompted greater investigation into the source and treatment of nocturnal asthma.

What Causes Nocturnal Asthma?

At one time it was thought nocturnal asthma was caused by the "wearing off" of medication during the night. Further research has shown that many factors are involved.

Adrenal Connection

It is well documented that there is a natural rhythm of the body in which many organs function differently during the night. The adrenal gland is no exception. During sleep the adrenal gland manufactures less cortisone and epinephrine causing a drop in their blood levels. Both of these substances are protective against asthma to a certain extent and the dip in blood levels may be one explanation for nocturnal asthma attacks.

Consider the Environment

Patients suffering nocturnal asthmatic attacks should look carefully at their bedrooms for sources of irritation. Potential allergens commonly found in bedrooms include feather pillows, animal dander, and dust mites. Simply using pillow and mattress covers may dramatically reduce nocturnal attacks. Other steps for removing allergens are detailed in chapter 6.

Reflux Connection

In chapter 10 the relationship between asthma and the stomach was discussed. Some doctors believe some nocturnal asthmatic attacks may be caused by reflux of stomach acid into the esophagus and throat where it may be aspirated into the bronchial tubes. Aggressive treatment of gastroesophageal reflux may reduce the frequency of nocturnal attacks.

Sinusitis and Nocturnal Asthma

The relationship between asthma and sinusitis was also discussed in chapter 10. Animal studies suggest that aspirating infected material from the sinuses into the lower throat and bronchial tubes may produce nocturnal asthma attacks. Although this effect has yet to be proven in patients with asthma, the strong possibility of a connection should reinforce vigorous treatment of sinusitis.

Other Factors in Nocturnal Asthma

Additional factors may also play a role in nocturnal asthma. It appears there is some cooling of airways at night. In asthmatics this change in temperature may be enough to produce asthma attacks. This mechanism also plays a role in exercise-induced asthma.

Some element in the nervous system may also be more active at night. The vagus nerve in the cholinergic nervous system is more active at night, and an increase in vagal tone may constrict the bronchial airways. In asthma patients that may increase the frequency of attacks.

Treating Nocturnal Asthma

Treating nocturnal asthma is based on the goal of achieving sufficient medication levels during sleep hours as well as eliminating environmental allergens. However, studies have shown that if patients are well controlled during the day, they will experience fewer and/or milder attacks at night. Asthma should always be regarded as a twenty-four-hour illness and treatment should not be directed solely at the nighttime hours.

Choosing Medication for Nocturnal Asthma

Many medications may be used to treat nocturnal asthma. More than one agent may be needed for patients with severe and frequent attacks.

B_2-agonists are available in long-acting forms both in aerosol (salmeterol) and tablet form (albuterol) that may be administered at night. By improving lung function and preventing nocturnal attacks, these agents may actually improve quality of sleep.

Theophylline in sustained-release forms allows once- or twice-a-day dosing and is suitable for nocturnal asthma treatment. The physician can time administration of this medication so peak blood levels are obtained during sleep. A common approach is one sustained-release preparation after the evening meal. Remember, theophylline blood levels can be measured and each sustained-release preparation is unique. One drawback of theophylline for nocturnal asthma is its potentially adverse effect of insomnia. Patients who limit their caffeine intake may reduce this effect.

Because overactivity of the cholinergic nervous system has been implicated in nocturnal asthma, anticholingeric agents have been administered at bedtime in patients with nocturnal asthma. High doses (ten puffs) of ipratropium bromide have been administered with conflicting results in several studies. At this time it does not appear that this agent is more effective than long-acting B_2-agonists for treating nocturnal asthma.

Patients with moderate to severe nocturnal asthma may need oral corticosteroids to control their symptoms. Studies of the timing of administration of this medication have shown dosing in early morning or evening does not achieve better control of nocturnal asthma. In these studies, patients who took steroid dosages at three P.M., however, significantly reduced the likelihood of nocturnal attacks.

Patients who continue to suffer nocturnal attacks despite aggressive therapy may need to awaken one hour before their usual nighttime attack to administer a short-acting B_2-agonist, an approach termed "therapeutic awakening."

Beta-Blockers and Asthma

A commonly prescribed group of medications, beta-blockers may produce severe, life-threatening asthmatic attacks. These medications are widely prescribed for multiple illnesses, including hypertension, cardiac arrhythmia, angina pectoris, glaucoma, and migraine.

The beta-receptors located in the lung (called beta-2 receptors), when active or stimulated, produce relaxation of the muscle surrounding the bronchial tubes, which widens the bronchial passage (bronchodilatation). If these receptors are blocked from receiving nerve input, the reverse effect (bronchoconstriction) results. This may have devastating effects on patients with underlying bronchial asthma. One theory for the nature of asthma postulated that the disease represented a "blockage" of the beta-receptor that was either inherited or established through acquired illness. It is easy to see why using beta-blockers in patients with asthma has produced fatal asthma attacks.

Beta-receptors are present in other organ systems such as the heart and circulation and are referred to as beta-1 receptors. Beta-blockers that affect beta-1 receptors more than beta-2 receptors are termed "selective." These medications vary in potency and duration. A number of the selective beta-blockers produce less blockade of lung receptors but there is still significant risk for exacerbating bronchial asthma. As a rule, all beta-blockers should be avoided by asthma patients.

Don't Forget Eyedrops!

Beta-blockers in the form of eyedrops are commonly used to treat glaucoma. Medication may be absorbed from the eye and delivered into the general blood circulation before reaching the bronchial tubes. Patients with bronchial asthma have suffered asthmatic attacks from beta-blockers introduced into the eye for treating glaucoma. Selective beta-blockers have been developed for glaucoma but may also produce bronchoconstriction. All patients with bronchial asthma should inform their ophthalmologists of their lung condition before treatment for glaucoma is initiated. In severe glaucoma cases where a beta-blocker is felt to be necessary, a selective agent should be used and the patient's airflows closely monitored.

Antidepressant Medication and B-Agonists

Monoamine oxidase (MAO) inhibitors are commonly prescribed for depression. These drugs inhibit the enzyme responsible for breaking down epinephrine released from the adrenal gland. When a B-adrenergic agonist is administered to patients receiving a MAO inhibitor there is a greater risk of adverse effects on the circulation, such as blood pressure elevation. This is more likely when the B-agonist is given by mouth or by injection since there is higher total-body absorption of the drug. By inhaling a B-agonist there is less chance of producing an adverse effect in a patient receiving a MAO inhibitor. When possible, an alternative antidepressant should be substituted in asthma patients to permit safe administration of a B-agonist. Patients who must receive both medications should be monitored closely for adverse circulatory effects.

Sedatives and Asthma

In asthma as in other chronic illnesses patients may experience increased levels of anxiety as well as sleeplessness. Requests for tranquilizers and sleeping pills are common. In patients with severe asthma, shortness of breath and fear of hospitalization may further heighten anxiety levels. Sleep may also be interrupted by asthmatic attacks.

Why to Avoid Tranquilizers and Sleeping Pills

All tranquilizers and sleeping pills affect the brain center that drives breathing. This reduces the activity of this vital center and causes more shallow breaths. Shallow breathing does not produce full expansion of the lung and results in lower oxygen levels. In patients with severe asthma, tranquilizers and sedatives may depress breathing which worsens attacks with possible life-threatening results. These patients should always avoid these agents.

Exceptions to the Rule

Patients with mild asthma and anxiety disorders such as panic attacks that require medication may receive tranquilizers. In these patients, close communication must be established between the primary physician and the psychiatrist prescribing the anxiety medication to ensure proper monitoring. This should include spirometry and a careful record of peak flows. Sleeping pills should generally be avoided even in patients with mild asthma other than for short-term use and only under careful physician supervision.

Oxygen Use in Asthma

When treating bronchial asthma, oxygen should be confined mainly to the emergency room and hospital setting because only in severe attacks do oxygen levels drop significantly. Besides, oxygen will not relieve bronchial constriction or in any way shorten an asthma attack.

There are some exceptions to this rule. Patients who have had severe, rapidly developing attacks in the past with low oxygen levels noted on admission to hospital and who are difficult to control, may keep an emergency oxygen cylinder at home. Patients with bronchial asthma and associated conditions like congestive heart failure or other heart diseases who might not tolerate *any* drop in oxygen level, may also keep a home emergency oxygen supply. Avoid routine use of oxygen in the home to treat uncomplicated bronchial asthma.

Premenstrual Asthma

Many women have noted premenstrual worsening of their asthma. Studies have demonstrated heightened sensitivity to various asthma triggers before menstruation. Hormonal treatment by injecting progesterone has been given to patients who suffer severe premenstrual exacerbations of their asthma. Additional measures that are helpful involve a step-by-step increase in medication possibly including a premenstrual increase in inhaled corticosteroid or a brief course of oral corticosteroid.

Just as in pregnancy, asthma varies from patient to patient prior to menstruation. Recording peak flows should help identify this form of asthma.

Sex and Asthma

The goal of achieving a normal lifestyle despite the presence of bronchial asthma certainly includes sexual activity. Sex should be regarded as healthy exercise to which many of the precautions concerning exercise-induced asthma can be applied.

Asthma medications do not affect sexual performance and can prevent asthmatic attacks that may be triggered by sexual activity. B-agonists should be taken prior to sex and cromolyn or nedocromil may be added if the B-agonist proves ineffective. Be sure you allow enough time for the medication to take effect. Avoiding allergens in the bedroom may be particularly important for sensitive patients to prevent attacks during sexual activity. Be sure to follow the steps for reducing dust mites in pillows, mattresses, and bed covers. Perfumes or colognes may also trigger attacks and should be avoided.

Patients and their sexual partners may want to discuss with the physician problems they have encountered during sex. Some patients may be more comfortable using positions that do not cause pressure to the chest. If asthma attacks have occurred during sex, reassurance to allay anxiety and additional steps to avoid further attacks should be discussed with your physician.

Asthma and Work Disability

Asthma is a frequent cause of work disability. In adults between the ages of eighteen and forty-four, asthma is second only to back problems as the leading cause of medical absence from work. A recent study of disability among adult asthmatics revealed that asthma frequently results in job changes and work duties that may cause a reduction in income.

How Is Work Disability Determined?

The variable nature of bronchial asthma makes determination of a work disability extremely difficult. Criteria for disability related to pulmonary disorders are based on measurements of lung function through pulmonary function tests. Patients with severe asthma may have symptom-free periods when lung function measurements exceed the criteria set by the American Medical Association. Therefore it is important to consider the frequency of your asthma attacks, what medications you need to control symptoms, and a reduction in day-to-day activities if you're being considered for work disability.

One important characteristic often present in patients disabled from bronchial asthma is dependence on oral corticosteroids to control their disease. Work disabled patients are often symptomatic despite maximum therapy with medication and are extremely limited in their activities. At least one study of disability in adult asthmatics has found a better correlation between disability and patient symptoms and the medications they need than with pulmonary function results. Guidelines combining all these factors need to be developed to better define disability in bronchial asthma.

CHAPTER 12

Future Considerations

New Medications

NEW and modified asthma medications are likely to improve treatment of bronchial asthma. Several medications already in general use in Canada and Europe are to be marketed in the United States in the near future. Many other medications are still being investigated. A new generation of asthma medications is likely to be available in the next year and will form an exciting period for both patients and the physicians involved in treating bronchial asthma.

Mediator Antagonists

Asthma mediator antagonists will soon offer a new generation of asthma medications. Asthma mediators are chemical substances produced by or normally stored in white blood cells like lymphocytes and are released during an attack. These mediators may stimulate or recruit other cells involved in an asthmatic reaction or have direct effects on the bronchial surface lining that lead to inflammation and swelling. Medications that inhibit or neutralize mediators like leukotrienes, platelet activating factor, and prostaglandins are currently under trial for treating asthma. These medications may be given by mouth or inhaled.

Zileuton

Leukotrienes are inflammatory substances produced by cells during asthma attacks. Zileuton is a medication that reduces leukotriene production by inhibiting an enzyme involved in its production. This medication has undergone extensive trials in the United States and should be the first of the "mediator antagonists" released in this country. Zileuton is taken by mouth, usually four times a day and appears to be well-tolerated. In patients with mild to moderate asthma, Zileuton appears to improve lung function and to reduce the frequency of asthma attacks. In one long-term study, patients treated with Zileuton used less B-agonist and required fewer courses of oral corticosteroids.

However, the chief role of Zileuton will be to prevent asthma attacks, not to treat acute asthma. A response may be noted after two to four weeks of treatment and maximal effect is achieved in one to four months. In about 2 percent of patients receiving Zileuton, abnormal liver blood tests have been reported. Patients receiving this medication should have periodic blood tests.

B_2-Agonists

Formoterol is a long-acting inhaled B_2-agonist aerosol that is already in use in Europe. Like salmeterol, it has a duration of twelve hours but appears to have a different mode of action. Formoterol appears to have faster onset than salmeterol and may be used for sudden attacks of asthma as well as for maintenance therapy.

Bambuterol is a drug that is converted by the body into another B-agonist, terbutaline. It is given by mouth and is effective for twenty-four hours. This once-a-day approach should be helpful, especially for patients with nocturnal asthma.

Inhaled Corticosteroids

Fluticasone

Fluticasone is a topical inhaled corticosteroid available in Europe that was recently released in the United States as a nasal spray. Fluticasone appears to be highly effective with low risk of total body absorption due to rapid breakdown. It is available in a "high-dose" form that allows patients to use fewer puffs per day and is available as a metered-dose inhaler and in a multidose dry powder inhaler. This highly potent agent appears to be extremely promising for treating bronchial asthma.

Budesonide

Another inhaled corticosteroid, budesonide, is also highly active topically and has been available in Europe and Canada for some time. It has been released in the United States as a nasal spray and should soon be available to treat asthma. Budesonide is available as a metered-dose inhaler and in low- and high-dose dry powder preparations.

Although there are few direct comparisons of the topical inhaled corticosteroids, budesonide appears to be highly potent with less total-body effects. It should offer an excellent alternative to currently available inhaled corticosteroids. Large studies comparing the inhaled corticosteroids in the treatment of bronchial asthma, however, have yet to be published.

Investigational Corticosteroids

Investigational agents in the inhaled steroid group undergoing trials at this time include mometasone and tipredane. Further data on these and additional agents should be available soon.

Immunomodulators

Medications called immunomodulators, that affect the immune response, are also being investigated. These agents would work along the same principle as corticosteroids that suppress the immune reaction.

Anticholinergic Agents

Oxitropium bromide is an anticholinergic bronchodilator similar to ipratropium bromide in its action. It appears to have a more potent effect and longer duration of action than ipratropium bromide.

Xanthines

Xanthines belong to the medication group that contains theophylline. Two agents, doxofylline and enprofylline have been studied and used in Europe. Doxofylline appears to have fewer side effects compared to theophylline and has been approved for use in Europe. The lower risk of adverse effects should reduce the need for blood level monitoring.

New Devices

Combination Sprays

Combination sprays containing both a B_2-agonist and an anticholinergic agent are likely to become increasingly available. The combination of these two bronchodilators appears to augment the effect produced by either if given alone. One spray that combines fenoterol and ipratropium bromide is available in Europe and has been marketed as Duovent. A combination spray containing albuterol and ipratropium bromide is under investigation in the United States.

Multidose Dry Powder Inhalers

Dry powder inhalers (DPIs) are likely to become increasingly available in multidose dispensers. Some are already available in Europe with "high-dose" preparations of B-agonists and inhaled corticosteroids. Currently, all DPIs are breath-activated but new designs are being developed. New DPIs would be triggered to release medication similar to metered-dose inhalers.

Metered-dose inhalers (MDIs) with new propellants that do not affect the ozone layer are also likely to be released before the end of this decade.

Breath-Activated Metered-Dose Inhalers

Because of the difficulty some patients have with timing inhalations of their medication, additional breath-activated devices will become available. The E-Z-V Inhalation Device has been developed by the Allen and Hanburys Division of Glaxo Inc., but has yet to gain FDA approval and may not be marketed in the United States. One advantage of this device over currently available breath-activated MDIs is an override button that could be pressed if the patient was unable to trigger the device by inhalation. This feature should be included in future breath-activated metered-dose inhalers.

The Next Generation

The next generation of asthma medications will most likely provide more sustained relief of symptoms with fewer puffs of medication. This should allow patients to use medication once or twice a day and still maintain control over their asthma. These new drugs will also be more specific antagonists of the chemicals that produce inflammation and bronchoconstriction.

The Environment

Increased environmental controls over outdoor and indoor air pollution will also improve quality of life of the patient with bronchial asthma as well as the entire population. Federal guidelines for outdoor pollution have been established under the Clean Air Act amended in 1990. It covers automobiles and industry and sets air quality standards. Regional compliance with these standards has yet to be achieved although progress has been made recently. Some states have passed laws with stricter standards that continue to tighten controls over automobile exhaust and the industrial combustion of fuels. Increased attention has also been directed at control of chlorofluorocarbon propellants that destroy the ozone layer. Although some progress has been made toward cleaner air, air pollution will continue to be a major source of lung disease well into the next century.

Greater attention must also be paid to "indoor pollution." This problem is now largely unregulated. Standards developed for outdoor pollution cannot be applied equally indoors. Fortunately, great strides have been made to restrict cigarette smoking. Further restrictions and ultimately a total ban on public smoking would be an important step toward reducing indoor and outdoor pollution as well as improving the general health of the entire population.

Every patient can be an active voice for improving the environment. Many organizations listed in appendix A can provide further information on how to be heard at the local, state, and federal levels.

Forming a Partnership Against Asthma with Your Physician

Although medications are likely to be better in the future, patients must maintain an active role in preventing asthma attacks, particularly by avoiding and reducing irritants and allergens in their home and work environments. If you have asthma, it is vital to acknowledge that you have a problem, then to deal with it by working with your physician. Too often, denying the problem only leads to unnecessary illness. This first step may be the most important in a series of measures you can take to avoid asthma attacks.

Other measures include an "early warning system" that relies on home peak flow measurements and close communication between patients and their physicians to prevent serious and even potentially fatal attacks. Patient education should be given a high priority by physicians and their staffs. Self-education should always be encouraged. Through dialogue and education patients can recognize when they must call for assistance, thereby avoiding the life-threatening tendency to "push through" a serious asthma attack on their own.

This partnership between patients and physicians, both working toward reducing the frequency and severity of attacks, can succeed in improving the quality of life for those who have asthma. Cooperation can also reduce the number of fatal asthma attacks that often could have been prevented by earlier recognition and treatment of this largely reversible disease.

Bibliography

Agata, H., A. Yomo, Y. Hanashiro et al. 1993. "Comparison of the MAST Chemiluminescent Assay System with RAST and Skin Tests in Allergic Children." *Annals of Allergy*, 70: 153–157.

Anderson, S.D., L.T. Rodwell, J. Du Toit, and I.H. Young. 1991. "Duration of Protection by Inhaled Salmeterol in Exercise-Induced Asthma." *Chest*, 100: 1254–1260.

Ballard, R.D. 1994. "Nocturnal Asthma: Potential Mechanisms and Current Therapy." *Clinical Pulmonary Medicine*, 1(5): 271–278.

Barnes, P. J. 1989. "A New Approach to the Treatment of Asthma." *The New England Journal of Medicine*, 321: 1517–1527.

———. 1994. "Blunted Perception and Death from Asthma." *The New England Journal of Medicine*, 330: 1383–1384.

Barnes, P.J., K.F. Chung, T.W. Evans, and S.G. Spiro. 1994. *Therapeutics in Respiratory Disease*. Edinburgh. Churchill Livingstone.

Bernstein, I.L. 1981. "Occupational Asthma." *Clinics in Chest Medicine*, 2(2): 255–272.

Bevelaqua, F.A. and F.V. Adams. 1993. "Pulmonary Disorders," in Eisenberg, M.G., R.L. Glueckauf, and H.H. Zaretsky (eds): *Medical Aspects of Disability* (325–341). New York. Springer.

Blanc, P.D. 1993. "Work Disability Among Adults with Asthma." *Chest*, 104: 1371–1377.

Britton, J., I. Pavord, K. Richards et al. 1994. "Dietary Magnesium, Lung Function, Wheezing, and Airway Hyper-reactivity in a Random Adult Population Sample." *Lancet*, 344: 357–362.

Burrows, B. and M.D. Lebowitz. 1992. "The B-Agonist Dilemma." *The New England Journal of Medicine*, 326: 560–561.

Check, W. A. and M. Kaliner. 1990. "Pharmacology and Pharmokinetics of Topical Corticosteroid Derivatives Used for Asthma Therapy." *American Review of Respiratory Disease*, 141: S44–S51.

D'Alonzo, G.E., S.I. Rennard, P.R. Ratner, and S.R. Findlay. 1992. "Twice-daily Inhaled Salmeterol as Maintenance Therapy for Asthma." *American Review of Respiratory Disease*, 145(4, pt 2): Abstract 65.

Dolovich, M., R. Ruffin, D. Corr, and M.T. Newhouse. 1983. "Clinical Evaluation of a Simple Demand Inhalation MDI Aerosol Delivery Device." *Chest*, 84: 36–41.

Engleberg, A. 1988. *The Respiratory System: Guides to the Evaluation of Permanent Impairment*. Chicago. American Medical Association.

Fiore, M.C., L.J. Baker, and S.M. Deeren. 1993. "Cigarette Smoking: The Leading Preventable Cause of Pulmonary Diseases," in Bone, R.C. *(ed)*: *Pulmonary and Critical Care Medicine.* St. Louis. Mosby.

Grossman, J. 1994. "The Evolution of Inhaler Technology." *Journal of Asthma*, 31(1): 55–64.

Guidelines for the Diagnosis and Management of Asthma. 1991. Washington, D.C.: U.S. Dept. of Health and Human Services (National Asthma Education Program). NIH Pub. No. 91–3042.

Haahtela, T., M. Jarvinen, T. Kava et al. 1994. "Effects of Reducing or Discontinuing Inhaled Budesonide in Patients with Mild Asthma." *The New England Journal of Medicine*, 331: 700–705.

Haas, F., S. Pasierski, N. Levine et al. 1987. "Effect of Aerobic Training On Forced Expiratory Airflow in Exercising Asthmatic Humans." *Journal of Applied Physiology*, 63: 1230–1235.

Hampson, N.B. and M.P. Mueller. 1994. "Reduction in Patient Timing Errors Using a Breath-activated Metered Dose Inhaler." *Chest*, 106(2): 462–465.

International Consensus Report on Diagnosis and Treatment of Asthma. 1992. Washington, D.C.: U.S. Dept. of Health and Human Services (International Asthma Management Project). NIH Pub. No. 92–3091.

Janson, C. et al. 1994. "Anxiety and Depression in Relation to Respiratory Symptoms and Asthma." *American Journal of Respiratory and Critical Care Medicine,* 149: 930–934.

Johansson, S.A., K.E. Andersson, R. Brattsand, et al. 1982. "Topical and Systemic Glucocorticoid Potencies of Budesonide and Beclomethasone Dipropionate in Man." *European Journal of Clinical Pharmacology,* 22: 523–529.

Kikuchi, Y., S. Okabe, and G. Tamura et al. 1994. "Chemosensitivity and Perception of Dyspnea in Patients with a History of Near-fatal Asthma." *The New England Journal of Medicine,* 330: 1329–1334.

Konig, P. 1988. "Inhaled Corticosteroids—Their Present and Future Role in the Management of Asthma." *The Journal of Allergy and Clinical Immunology,* 82(2): 297–306.

Lee, N., G. Rachelefsky, and R.H. Kobayashi et al. 1991. "Efficacy and Safety of Albuterol Administered by Power-Driven Nebulizer (PDN) Versus Metered-Dose Inhaler (MDI) with Aerochamber and Mask in Infants and Young Children with Acute Asthma." *Journal of Allergy and Clinical Immunology,* 87 (Suppl.) (1, pt. 2): 307.

Management of Asthma During Pregnancy. 1993. Washington, D.C.: U.S. Dept. of Health and Human Services (Report of the Working Group on Asthma and Pregnancy). NIH Pub. No. 93–3279A.

McCallum, R.W. 1994. "Cisapride for the Treatment of Nocturnal Heartburn in Patients with Gastroesophageal Reflux Disease." *Today's Therapeutic Trends,* 11(4): 187–201.

Newhouse, M.T. 1993. "Pulmonary Drug Targeting with Aerosols. Principles and Clinical Applications in Adults and Children." *The American Journal of Asthma & Allergy for Pediatricians,* 7(1): 23–35.

Newman, S.P., G. Woodman, S.W. Clarke, and M.A. Sackner. 1986. "Effect of InspirEase on the Deposition of Metered-Dose Aerosols in the Human Respiratory Tract." *Chest,* 89: 551–556.

O'Connor, B.J., S. Uden, T.J. Carty et al. 1994. "Inhibitory Effect of UK, 74505, a Potent and Specific Oral Platelet Activating Factor (PAF) Receptor Antagonist, on Airway and Systemic Responses to Inhaled PAF in Humans." *American Journal of Respiratory and Critical Care Medicine*, 150: 35–40.

Pearlman, D.S., P. Chervinsky, C. Laforce et al. 1992. "A Comparison of Salmeterol with Albuterol in the Treatment of Mild-to-Moderate Asthma." *The New England Journal of Medicine*, 327: 1420–1425.

Petrie, G.R. 1993. "Bambuterol: Effective in Nocturnal Asthma." *Respiratory Medicine*, 87: 581–585.

Rau, J.L., Jr. 1994. *Respiratory Care Pharmacology*. St. Louis. Mosby.

Samet, J.M. and M.J. Utell. 1993. "Air Pollution," in Bone, R.C. (ed): *Pulmonary and Critical Care Medicine*. St. Louis. Mosby.

Shirakawa, T., L. Airong, M. Dubowitz et al. 1994. "Assocation Between Atopy and Variants of the B Subunit of the High-Affinity Immunoglobulin E Receptor. *Nature Genetics*, 7(2): 125–129.

Sorkness, R., J.J. Clough, W.L. Castleman, and R.F Lemanske, Jr. 1994. "Virus-induced Airway Obstruction and Parasympathetic Hyperresponsiveness in Adult Rats." *American Journal of Respiratory and Critical Care Medicine*, 150: 28–34.

Spector, S.L., L.J. Smith, M. Glass et al. 1994. "Effect of 6 Weeks of Therapy with Oral Doses of ICI 204,219, a Leukotriene D_4 Receptor Antagonist in Subjects With Bronchial Asthma." *American Journal of Repiratory and Critical Care Medicine*, 150: 618–623.

Spitzer, W.O., S. Suissa, and P. Ernst et al. 1992. "The Use of B-Agonists and the Risk of Death and Near Death from Asthma." *The New England Journal of Medicine*, 326: 502–506.

Thompson, J., T. Irvine, K. Grathwohl, and B. Roth. 1994. "Misuse of Metered-dose Inhalers in Hospitalized Patients." *Chest*, 105(3): 715–717.

Turkeltaub, P.C. 1994. "Deaths Associated with Allergenic Extracts." *FDA Medical Bulletin*, 24(1): 7.

Vanzieleghem, M.A. and E.F. Juniper. 1987. "A Comparison of Budesonide and Beclomethasone Dipropionate Nasal Aerosols in Ragweed-induced Rhinitis." *Journal of Allergy and Clinical Immunology*, 79: 887–892.

Weiss, K. B., P.J. Gergen, and T. A. Hodgson. 1992. "An Economic Evaluation of Asthma in the United States." *The New England Journal of Medicine*, 326: 862–866.

How to Get More Help

Telephone Hotlines

American Lung Association
> 1-800-LUNG USA
> Information on this nationwide organization and how to reach your local chapter.

Asthma and Allergy Foundation Patient Information Line
> 1-800-7-ASTHMA
> General information, publications, videos, and referrals to physicians.

Asthma Information Line
> 1-800-822-ASMA
> Provides written materials on asthma and allergies. Operates 24 hours a day.

Lung Line
> 1-800-222-LUNG
> Staffed by registered nurses and managed by National Jewish Center for Immunology and Respiratory Medicine. Provides information on all types of lung disease.

Newsletters

Asthma and Allergy Advocate
    Publisher: American Academy of Allergy and Immunology
    Address: 611 East Wells Street
                 Milwaukee, WI 53202
    Contains practical advice for patients with asthma and allergies.

Asthma Update
    Publisher: David C. Jamison
    Address: 123 Monticello Avenue
                 Annapolis, MD 21401
    Informative publication with articles about new developments, practical
    advice for patients and parents of children with asthma, and available
    resources.

Air Currents
    Publisher: Allen & Hanbury's, Division of Glaxo
    Address: Respiratory Institute
                 5 Moore Drive
                 Research Triangle Park, NC 27709
    Reports on new trends in asthma as well as general information on respi-
    ratory disease.

The MA Report
    Publisher: Asthma and Allergy Network (AAN)/
                 Mothers of Asthmatics, Inc.
    Address: 3554 Chain Bridge Road, Suite 200
                 Fairfax, VA 22030
    Telephone: 703-385-4403
                 1-800-878-4403
    Monthly with practical information for families of children with asthma.
    Patients or parents may write in questions that are answered by a team of
    specialists.

New Directions
> Publisher: National Jewish Center for Immunology and Respiratory
> Medicine
> Address: 1400 Jackson Street
> Denver, CO 80206

Informative publication focused on new developments in respiratory disease.

Audiovisual Aids

Managing Childhood Asthma
> Publisher: Allergy and Asthma Network/Mothers of Asthmatics, Inc.
> Address: 3554 Chain Bridge Road, Suite 200
> Fairfax, VA 22030

Instructive video focused on the asthmatic child functioning normally in school, at play, and in the home.

Living With It (Asthma)
> Publisher: St. John's Hospital
> Long Beach Memorial Medical Center
> 2801 Atlantic Avenue
> Long Beach, CA 90801-1428

Aerobics for Asthmatics
> Publisher: Aerobics for Asthmatics, Inc.
> Address: 10301 Georgia Avenue, Suite 306
> Silver Spring, MD 20902

Exercise video designed by swimmer and Olympic gold medalist Nancy Hogshead in cooperation with Stanley I. Wolf, M.D., and Kathy L. Lampl, M.D. Available through Allergy and Asthma Network/Mothers of Asthmatics, Inc.

Allergy Control Begins at Home
        Publisher: Allergy Control Products, Inc.
        Address: 96 Danbury Road
                            Ridgefield, CT 06866
Informative video containing detailed scientific discussion of the biology
and living habits of dust mites as well as steps to reduce exposure.
Includes commentary by experts from The Asthma and Allergic Diseases
Center at the University of Virginia.

Pamphlets

A Patient's Guide to Asthma
        Author: Fred Leffert, M.D.
        Publisher: Allen & Hanbury's, Division of Glaxo
        Address: 5 Moore Drive
                            Research Triangle Park, NC 27709

Asthma, Facts About (ALA #0052)
About Lungs and Lung Diseases (ALA #0001)
Controlling Asthma (ALA #1125)
There Are Solutions for the Student with Asthma (ALA #0083)
What Happens When a Child Has Asthma (ALA #0069)
Occupational Asthma (Facts About: Lung Hazards on the Job) (ALA #0211)
Asthma...At My Age? (ALA #1551)
Peak Flow Meters, Facts About (ALA #0427)
Childhood Asthma, A Matter of Control (ALA #6012)
Home Control of Allergies and Asthma (ALA #3512)
        Publisher: American Lung Association
        Address: 1740 Broadway
                            New York, NY 10019-4374

Becoming Close
        Publisher: National Jewish Center
        Address: 1400 Jackson Street
                            Denver, CO 80206
Sexual concerns of patients with respiratory disease.

Sneezeless Landscaping
    Publisher: ALA of Oregon
    Address: 1776 SW Madison
                 Portland, OR 97205
    Describes plants that may cause allergic reactions; offers alternatives for your garden.

The User's Guide to Peak Flow Monitoring
    Author: Guillermo Mendoza, M.D.
    Publisher: Allergy and Asthma Network/Mothers of Asthmatics, Inc.
    Address: 3554 Chain Bridge Road, Suite 200
                 Fairfax, VA 22030
    Describes how to use peak flow meter. Information for children and adults.

Booklets

The Asthma Handbook (ALA #4002) (Spanish language version ALA #4003)
    Publisher: American Lung Association
    Address: 1740 Broadway
                 New York, NY 10019-4374
    A concise, helpful 24-page handbook for adult patients with asthma.

Let's Talk About Asthma. A Guide for Teens (ALA #1552)
    Author: Joyce Baldwin
    Publisher: American Lung Association
    Address: 1740 Broadway
                 New York, NY 10019-4374
    Informative booklet addressing concerns of teenagers with asthma.

The Asthma Organizer
    Author: Nancy Sander, Debra Scherrer, and Martha White, M.D.
    Publisher: Allergy and Asthma Network/Mothers of Asthmatics, Inc.
    Address: 3554 Chain Bridge Road, Suite 200
                 Fairfax, VA 22030
    Informative notebook for planning a daily strategy for managing and monitoring asthma. Available in Spanish or English.

Books

Asthma and Exercise

Author: Nancy Hogshead and Gerald S. Couzens
Publisher: Allergy and Asthma Network/Mothers of Asthmatics, Inc.
Address: 3554 Chain Bridge Road, Suite 200
            Fairfax, VA 22030

Detailed recommendations for children and adults with asthma on exercise and participation in athletics.

Children with Asthma: A Manual for Parents

Author: Thomas Plaut, M.D.
Publisher: Pedi Press, Inc.
Length: 268 pages

Highly comprehensive; valuable for parents of asthmatic children.

Cooking for the Allergic Child

Author: Judy Moyer
Publisher: Grove Printing
Length: 314 pages

Written by the mother of an allergic child. Contains more than 300 recipes designed for the entire family and for all occasions. Nutritional information included.

Luke Has Asthma, Too

Author: Allison Rodgers
Publisher: Waterfront Books
Length: 29 pages

Illustrated short story for children aged 3–7, aimed at reassuring both the asthmatic child and parents. General information on medication, breathing exercises, and what happens if hospitalization is needed.

Winning Over Asthma

Author: Eileen Dolan Savage

Publisher: Pedipress, Inc.

Address: 125 Red Gate Lane

             Amherst, MA 01002

Length: 28 pages

Illustrated short book about Graham, a five-year-old with asthma. Emphasizes asthma can be controlled with medication and a teamwork approach among doctor, patient, and family.

School Materials

Managing Asthma: A Guide for Schools

Publisher: National Asthma Education and Prevention Program

Address: National Heart, Lung and Blood Institute

             P.O. Box 30105

             Bethesda, MD 20824-0105

Open Airways For Schools

Publisher: American Lung Association

Address: Open Airways For Schools

             P.O. Box 1036

             Evans City, PA 16033

Telephone: 1-800-292-5542

Inexpensive program developed and evaluated at Columbia University's College of Physicians and Surgeons for elementary schools. Teaching materials include curriculum, instructor's guide, poster flip chart, and reproducible handouts for children and parents. Each package designed to serve an entire school and may be reused.

Asthma In The School: Improving Control With Peak Flow Monitoring
   Author: Guillermo Mendoza, M.D., Mary Kay Garcia, R.N.
                and Mary Collins, M.A.
   Publisher: Allergy and Asthma Network/Mothers of Asthmatics, Inc.
   Address: 3554 Chain Bridge Road, Suite 200
                Fairfax, VA 22030
   Practical guide for the school nurse to help students monitor their asthma.

National Societies

Allergy and Asthma Network/Mothers of Asthmatics, Inc. (AAN/MA)
   3554 Chain Bridge Road, Suite 200
   Fairfax, VA 22030
   Telephone: 1-800-878-4403
   This health organization was originally Mothers of Asthmatics and was
   founded in 1985 by Nancy Sander. AAN/MA provides accurate, up-to-date
   information for patients and their families to support a greater understanding of allergy and asthma. AAN/MA has written *A Bill of Rights for
   Children with Allergies and Asthma* endorsed by the American Academy of
   Pediatrics and the American Academy of Allergy and Immunology. Mem-
   bership includes subscription to the monthly newsletter *The MA Report* as
   well as discounts on allergy and asthma products and publications. List of
   publications, videos, and other informative materials provided by this
   organization may be obtained by calling the above number.

American Academy of Allergy and Immunology
   611 East Wells Street
   Milwaukee, WI 53202
   Professional society of allergists and related specialists publishes *Asthma
   and Allergy Advocate* for patients and the *Journal of Allergy and Clinical
   Immunology* for physicians.

American College of Allergy and Immunology
    800 East Northwest Highway, Suite 1080
    Palatine, IL 60067
    Professional society of allergists and related specialists. Publishes *Annals of Allergy and Immunology* for physicians.

American Lung Association (ALA)
    1740 Broadway
    New York, NY 10019-4374
    Telephone: 212-315-8700
    ALA is a highly informative national organization with local chapters throughout the U.S. Publishes numerous pamphlets and booklets on all types of lung disease as well as audiovisual aids, posters, and signs. ALA also sponsors programs for the lay public on lung disease, smoking cessation, support groups, and asthma camps. One important function is to raise funds and sponsor research into lung diseases. Locate your local chapter by calling 1-800-LUNG USA or check your telephone directory. Your local chapter should provide information on regional support groups and asthma camps.

American Thoracic Society (ATS)
    1740 Broadway
    New York, NY 10019-4374
    ATS is the medical branch of the American Lung Association. Besides many other scientific activities, ATS/ALA has initiated the Asthma Research Campaign designed to promote multidisciplinary research aimed at producing a major advance in preventing and treating asthma. ATS also publishes *American Journal of Respiratory and Critical Care Medicine.*

Asthma and Allergy Foundation of America (AAFA)
    1125 15th Street NW, Suite 502
    Washington, DC 20005
    Telephone: 1-800-7-ASTHMA
    National organization sponsoring educational programs for patients with asthma and allergies as well as promoting research and asthma support groups. AAFA publishes the newsletter *Advance.*

National Asthma Education and Prevention Program (NAEP)
National Heart, Lung and Blood Institute (NHLBI)
>P.O. Box 30105
>Bethesda, MD 20824-0105
>Telephone: 301-251-1222
>Established in 1989 by NHLBI, NAEP was formed to increase awareness of asthma as a serious chronic disease and to disseminate information that ensures proper diagnosis and treatment. In 1991, NAEP published *Guidelines for the Diagnosis and Management of Asthma* for physicians and other health care providers. NAEP also publishes educational material for patients and families including *Your Asthma Can Be Controlled: Accept Nothing Less*. These and other pamphlets on asthma in English or Spanish may be obtained by calling or writing.

Asthma Research Council
>12 Pembridge Square
>London W2 4EH
>United Kingdom
>A U.K. organization comparable to the American Lung Association, with branches in major cities.

The National Institute of Allergy and Infectious Diseases (NIAID)
>Building 31, Room 7A50
>9000 Rockville Pike
>Bethesda, MD 20205
>Division of the National Institutes of Health (NIH). NIAID publishes several pamphlets on allergy that patients may obtain by writing to the above address.

Referral Centers

National Jewish Center for Immunology and Respiratory Medicine
   1400 Jackson Street
   Denver, CO 80206
   Telephone: 1-800-423-8891
   National Jewish Center is a world-renowned medical center for research
   and evaluation and treatment of pulmonary diseases including asthma.
   Patients of any age may be evaluated either as inpatients (if they need
   urgent hospital care) or as outpatients. Length of stay may vary from days
   to weeks depending on individual needs. Evaluations are thorough and
   combine several disciplines, including allergy, immunology, and pul-
   monology. Emphasis on patient education and self monitoring as well as
   incorporating family into patient-support mechanism. Reports sent
   promptly to referring physicians.

Alfred I. duPont Institute Asthma Program
   Wilmington, DE
   Telephone: 302-651-4000
   Comprehensive program for children with severe asthma that combines
   inpatient evaluation and outpatient patient and family therapy.

Obtaining Allergy Supplies

Allergy Control Products, Inc.
   Address: 96 Danbury Road
                Ridgefield, CT 06877
   Telephone: 1-800-422-DUST
   Mail-order company offering a comprehensive list of products incorpo-
   rated into an educational brochure. Products include several types of
   mattress and pillow covers, HEPA air filters and vacuum cleaners, anti-
   dust mite sprays and carpet treatments. Catalog includes washable
   stuffed animals as well as a dust analysis kit for evaluating your own
   environment.

Bio-Tech Health Systems, Ltd.
    Address: P.O. Box 18398
                  Chicago, IL 60618
    Telephone: 1-800-621-5545
    Mail-order company providing wide selection of allergy products. Catalog includes hints on preventing allergy as well as wide selection of mattress and pillow covers, HEPA air filters and vacuum cleaners, nebulizers, peak flow meters, spacers and many other materials. Order form includes a certificate of "medical necessity" that may allow insurance reimbursement.

Envirahealth Inc.
    Address: 34 South Broadway, 7th Floor Suite
                  White Plains, N.Y. 10601
    Telephone: 1-800-877-7772
    Informative company provides full line of allergy products including HEPA air purifiers and vacuum cleaners, bedding protectors, humidifiers, dehumidifiers, cleaning products for pets (Allerpet), anti-dust mite powder (Acarosan), and home dust analysis kits. Extremely helpful service; will obtain any allergy product.

Environmental Health Shopper
    Address: P.O. Box 239
                  Fate, Texas 75132
    Telephone: 1-800-447-1100
    Mail-order company provides many allergy products. Catalog includes water filtration systems, water testing kits, mattress and pillow covers, cleaning products, and personal care products.

Glossary

Acaracide: Agent that kills mites that could be used in the home to eradicate dust mites.

Acetylcholine: Chemical substance stored in nerve endings of parasympathetic nervous system released when nerves are stimulated, producing a response.

Aerosol: Fine mist that can be inhaled; may be produced by metered-dose inhaler or nebulizer.

Adrenergic: Refers to sympathetic nervous system and its nerve fibers and receptors. Stimulating these receptors in the bronchial tubes produces bronchial muscle relaxation, resulting in opening of the bronchial tubes.

Agonist: Drug or agent with an affinity for corresponding nerve receptor that may stimulate the receptor to produce its effect. I.e.: a B(beta)-agonist attaches to beta receptor producing relaxation of bronchial lining muscle.

Airway hyperreactivity: Asthma characteristic in which bronchial tubes react to substances or stimuli by closing or constricting, a reaction that does not occur in non-asthmatics.

Allergen: Substance producing allergic reaction, i.e.: airborne pollen.

Allergy: Hypersensitivity to specific substance. When an allergic person is exposed to an offending substance a "reaction" occurs that may take several forms (tearing of eyes, sneezing, wheezing) varying from person to person.

Alveoli: Tiny air sacs that make up lung tissue where the exchange of oxygen and carbon dioxide occurs.

Anaphylaxis: Extremely severe allergic reaction involving the total body. Often characterized by "closing" of the throat and constriction of bronchial tubes. May result in collapse of body's circulation (shock) and death.

Atelectasis: Lung condition in which tiny air sacs or alveoli are collapsed.

Atopy: Condition of being allergic, often used interchangeably with "allergy."

Autonomic nervous system: Body involuntary control system that maintains many functions. Divided into parasympathetic and sympathetic branches.

Beta-agonist: Medication stimulating nerve receptors that produce bronchial tube dilatation.

Beta-receptor: Nerve ending site responsible for bronchial tube condition.

Bronchial tubes: Air passages of the lung through which air exchange takes place. The asthmatic reaction takes place in these tubes.

Bronchiectasis: Condition where infection has damaged the bronchial tube wall producing chronic cough and production of infected sputum. Wheezing may also occur and may be confused with asthma.

Bronchoconstriction: Narrowing or closing of bronchial tubes. One characteristic of asthmatic reaction.

Bronchodilatation: Opening or widening of bronchial tubes. Reverse of bronchoconstriction.

Bronchodilator: Agent or medication producing bronchodilatation.

Bronchoscopy: Procedure in which lighted scope called bronchoscope is introduced into lungs through bronchial tubes. Usually done to investigate certain lung diseases.

Bronchospasm: Another term for narrowing of bronchial airways. Same as bronchoconstriction.

Candidiasis: Fungal infection caused by common yeast called *candida*. May occur in the mouth in patients with poor oral hygiene who use corticosteroid spays. May be prevented with simple precautions and treated with antifungal medication.

Capillaries: Tiny blood vessels found in walls of alveoli in lung and other parts of body. In the lung vessels pick up oxygen and release carbon dioxide.

Carbon dioxide (C0$_2$): Waste product of body metabolism. Gas excreted by lung in exhalation.

CFC: Abbreviation for chlorofluorocarbons, chemical aerosols currently powering metered-dose inhalers. Known to be harmful to the ozone layer.

Cholinergic: Agent or medication stimulating parasympathetic nervous system. In the lung causes contraction of bronchial muscle producing bronchoconstriction.

Chromosome: Structure within body cells that contains genes.

Corticosteroid: Group of medications derived from adrenal gland.

Cystic Fibrosis: Hereditary childhood lung disease characterized by cough, thick mucus, and recurrent lung infections. Wheezing may also occur and cause confusion with asthma diagnosis.

DPI: Dry powder inhaler abbreviation.

Emphysema: Lung disease in which walls of air sacs are destroyed and supporting structure of bronchial tubes is weakened. Emphysema may be confused with asthma due to presence of wheezing.

Endoscope: Flexible, lighted instrument for examining internal organs. See, bronchoscope.

Eosinophil: A white blood cell associated with allergic reactions; often involved in asthma.

Ergometer: Instrument for measuring amount of work or energy the body uses.

Expiratory: Relating to breathing out or exhaling.

Fiberoptic: Fine glass fibers that transmit images in instruments for examining internal organs (endoscopes).

Freon: See, CFC.

Gastroesophageal: Relating to upper digestive system, including feeding passage (esophagus) and stomach.

HEPA: High-efficiency particulate air purifier. HEPA filters can be used in room air purifiers, central ventilation systems, and vacuum cleaners.

Histamine: Chemical substance contained in MAST cells and other white blood cells. When histamine is released from these cells, may cause many features of allergic reaction.

Humidification: Addition of moisture to air. May be used to loosen dried secretion in sinuses or bronchial tubes.

Humoral: Relating to substance produced in body that acts at a specific site; i.e.: production of antibodies by immune system.

Hyperinflated: Lung condition in which they are overexpanded. May occur in asthma when inhaled air is "trapped" by narrowed bronchial tubes.

Hyperreactivity: Condition of increased sensitivity or irritability, a feature of bronchial tubes in asthma.

Hyperresponsiveness: See, hyperreactivity.

Immunoglobulin: Protein substance produced by immune system in response to body being invaded by foreign substance (allergen, bacteria). Several types are manufactured depending on the invader.

Immunoglobulin E: IgE, type of immunoglobulin produced when sensitive individual is exposed to allergens. Blood level of IgE may identify presence of allergy in some individuals. IgE is involved in allergic reaction that allows allergy chemicals to be released from storage cells.

Immunotherapy: Allergy treatment also known as "desensitization" or "allergy shots." Injections of extracts of allergy substances are given in increasing strengths over time.

Intranasal: Refers to application of medication into nasal passages.

Intravenous: Injecting medication directly into a vein.

Intubation: Placing breathing tube into windpipe, performed when artificial or mechanical respiration is needed.

Lymphocyte: White blood cell commonly involved in immune reactions. T lymphocytes are involved in cellular reactions; B lymphocytes are responsible for production of antibodies.

Mast cells: Body cells contain chemicals that are mediators of asthma and allergy reactions. These cells are distributed throughout the body and are commonly found on the surfaces of the nose, throat, and bronchial tubes. When these cells are destroyed their chemical contents are released and allergy and asthma reactions occur.

Mediator: Chemical substance that produces a body reaction when released.

Metered-dose inhaler (MDI): Hand-held applicator that dispenses liquid asthma medication in an aerosol medium for inhalation.

Methacholine: Cholinergic drug that may produce bronchoconstriction when administered to asthmatics. Often used in bronchial challenge testing to demonstrate presence or absence of reactive airways.

Mucosa: Mucous membrane covering inner surface of many structures in the body including nose and bronchial tubes. This delicate bronchial lining swells and becomes inflamed in an asthmatic attack.

Myopathy: Muscle abnormality possibly characterized by weakness and atrophy. Potential adverse effect of systemic corticosteroids.

Nebulizer: Device dispensing liquid medication as fine mist that is inhaled. Devices vary in size of particles they dispense.

Neurotransmitter: Chemical substance that facilitates conduction of nerve impulses.

Neutrophil: Type of white blood cell often involved in immune reactions.

NSAID: Abbreviation for NonSteroidal Anti-Inflammatory Drug.

Ostia: Openings in various canals or tubes throughout body. I.e.: nasal and sinus passages.

O-T-C: Over-the-counter. Medications sold this way do not need a physician prescription.

Oximeter: Device measuring saturation or enrichment of blood with oxygen.

Oxygen: Gas needed for life-sustaining activities of body. Taken up by red blood cells within walls of alveoli.

Particulates: Fine airborne particles (soot) produced by fuel combustion. Component of air pollution.

Polypectomy: Surgical procedure to remove polyps from various body locations including nose and sinuses. Recent advances in technology may allow polyp removal by endoscopic surgery.

Prokinetic: Characteristic of certain medications that increase forward motility of digestive tract. May be used to treat gastroesophageal reflux.

Pulmonologist: Internist with specialized training in lung diseases. After completing required training physician may take certifying examination in pulmonary disease given by American Board of Internal Medicine.

RAST: Abbreviation for radioallergosorbent test, blood test that can identify allergy to specific substances. Measures amount of IgE manufactured by body against specific allergens. Alternative to allergy scratch tests.

Reflux: Backward flow. Term commonly describing regurgitation of stomach contents into feeding passage (esophagus).

Rhinitis: Inflammation of nasal membranes or lining. Rhinitis may be allergic or nonallergic.

Scratch test: Allergy test in which skin is scratched and drop of allergen is placed on scratched area. Alternative is prick test in which allergen is placed on skin and skin is pricked with needle.

Spirometer: Instrument used to measure air capacity of lungs. May also be equipped to measure speed of air movement.

Spirometry: Testing with spirometer. May be called "Pulmonary Function Test."

Sputum: Material coughed up from lungs; also "phlegm." Consisting of mucus, cells, and debris resulting from bacteria.

Symptomatology: Aggregate of symptoms from disease.

Systemic: Term referring to entire body. Often describes how a medication is given. In contrast to "local" medication given at specific site, systemic drugs are taken by mouth or intravenously and pass through entire body.

Tomography: X-ray technique allowing sections of a structure to be visualized in detail.

Trachea: Main air passage or windpipe beginning below voice box (larynx) and ends when it divides into the right and left main bronchial tubes. Trachea is considered one of the "large airways."

Urticaria: Skin eruption of hives. Usually represents systemic allergic reaction.

Vagus: Major nerve with parasympathetic (cholinergic) fibers distributed to bronchial tubes. Stimulating these nerves may cause constriction of bronchial tubes. Anticholinergic medications that block vagal impulses may be bronchodilatators.

Index